Immunity

IMMUNITY

William E. Paul, MD

JOHNS HOPKINS UNIVERSITY PRESS | BALTIMORE

Note to the Reader: This book is not meant to substitute for medical care, and treatment should not be based solely on its contents. Instead, treatment must be developed in a dialogue between the individual and his or her physician. This book has been written to help with that dialogue.

Drug dosage: The author and publisher have made reasonable efforts to determine that the selection of drugs discussed in this text conform to the practices of the general medical community. The medications described do not necessarily have specific approval by the U.S. Food and Drug Administration for use in the diseases for which they are recommended. In view of ongoing research, changes in governmental regulation, and the constant flow of information relating to drug therapy and drug reactions, the reader is urged to check the package insert of each drug for any change in indications and dosage and for warnings and precautions. This is particularly important when the recommended agent is a new and/or infrequently used drug.

Contributions provided by Dr. William Paul to the book were written in a personal capacity and do not necessarily represent the opinions or endorsement of the National Institutes of Health, Department of Health and Human Services, or the Federal Government.

© 2015 William E. Paul
All rights reserved. Published 2015
Printed in the United States of America on acid-free paper
9 8 7 6 5 4 3 2 1

Johns Hopkins University Press
2715 North Charles Street
Baltimore, Maryland 21218-4363
www.press.jhu.edu

Library of Congress Cataloging-in-Publication Data

Paul, William E., author.
    Immunity / William E. Paul.
        p. ; cm.
    Includes bibliographical references and index.
    ISBN 978-1-4214-1801-8 (hardcover : alk. paper) — ISBN 1-4214-1801-0 (hardcover : alk. paper) — ISBN 978-1-4214-1802-5 (electronic) — ISBN 1-4214-1802-9 (electronic)
    I. Title.
    [DNLM: 1. Immune System Phenomena. 2. Immunity. 3. Immune System Diseases—immunology. QW 540]
    RC582
    616.07'9—dc23   2015002906

A catalog record for this book is available from the British Library.

Special discounts are available for bulk purchases of this book. For more information, please contact Special Sales at 410-516-6936 or specialsales@press.jhu.edu.

Johns Hopkins University Press uses environmentally friendly book materials, including recycled text paper that is composed of at least 30 percent post-consumer waste, whenever possible.

31.67

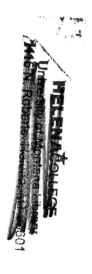

To Marilyn

Nothing is more powerful than an idea whose time has come.

—paraphrased from Victor Hugo (*On résiste à l'invasion des armées; on ne résiste pas à l'invasion des idées*), *Histoire d'un crime*

Contents

Preface

When the immune system is acting normally, it protects us against infectious diseases and helps us to resist cancer. When boosted by vaccines, its power is immense. Vaccination is the only medical intervention that has led to complete eradication of a disease—two, in fact. Through vaccination, the immune system has eliminated smallpox and rinderpest from the planet.

But there are dangerous aspects of immunity as well. They include not only well-known autoimmune diseases such as type 1 diabetes mellitus, multiple sclerosis, the inflammatory bowel diseases, thyroiditis, rheumatoid arthritis, and systemic lupus erythematosus but also atherosclerosis, cirrhosis of the liver, type 2 diabetes, and other inflammatory diseases.

My goal in writing this book is to introduce both general readers and potential students of immunology to this fascinating subject and to aid them in understanding how the immune system carries out its remarkable protective functions and how at the same time can be so dangerous.

Immunology is one of the powerhouses driving advances in twenty-first-century medicine. Understanding how immunity works will give readers tools to make informed decisions about their health and to exercise informed judgment in the political arena—in support of or in opposition to laws regarding vaccination or quarantine, for example. This understanding will also help readers evaluate the various, often fantastical, claims advanced in many popular books and articles. A deeper understanding of immunity will allow an appreciation of the great value of vaccines and will counter many of the assertions of those opposed to vaccination.

Readers will quickly realize that the road to modern immunology was by no means a superhighway. The twists and turns are many, but they represent some of the best of modern science—and they make a fascinating narrative. I have been an active player in this field since my postdoctoral fellowship in the 1960s and have witnessed the great advances and even contributed to some of them. I intersperse my own experiences throughout the book, both to give a sense of a "life in science" but also to allow a description of the actual experiments, warts and all, that contributed to this progress. While I have made every effort to be certain my recounting of immunology is factually correct, I have, of course, placed emphasis on particular areas and stressed the significance of certain contributions. Other authors might have approached the story of immunology somewhat differently and emphasized areas that I have not, perhaps downplaying accomplishments to which I have attributed great significance. I believe this is inevitable in a field as complex and as rich in accomplishment as immunology.

Immunity begins with an overview of the critical importance of immunology to our lives and a description of how an immune response to a typical infectious agent progresses. It illustrates the various "weapons" the immune system uses to protect us. This section then lays out three organizing laws of immunology. These are not like laws of physics but rather like laws that we make to govern our behavior; these laws can be broken, but there is a price to pay, often a very steep one. I close part one with a description of my personal introduction to immunology.

Part two considers in depth the first of the laws, universality. This part's central theme is provided in chapter 7, which describes immunology's "eureka" concept: that each newly minted lymphocyte has a unique specificity and that the vast range of specific responses the immune system can develop is due to an extremely large number of lymphocytes, each with the capacity to mount a distinct immune response.

In part three I develop the concept of tolerance, which states that while it is possible to make immune responses specific for virtually any molecular structure of appropriate size, one set of structures is largely exempt from such responses: the structures found in the individual mounting an immune response. That is to say, the individual generally (but unfortunately not always) does not make immune responses against his or her own tissues. Avoiding self-responses is so critical that several mechanisms have evolved either to eliminate the cells that would make such responses or, if that fails, to control these responses. An important component of this control is mediated through the action of a specialized set of cells called regulatory T cells (Tregs).

Part four deals with the third of the laws, appropriateness. The need for appropriateness is based on the differences in the niches within our bodies that different infectious agents attack and on the differences in the nature of those attacks. Responses to distinct infectious attacks must be suited to the particular assault. An optimal immune response against a viral infection of the lung will need to be quite different from a protective response to a parasitic worm infecting the gastrointestinal tract. That is, the immune system must recognize the nature of the threat and develop a response well suited to deal with it. The immunity that develops must be qualitatively and quantitatively appropriate.

Part five introduces the reader to a much older immune system than the one that is the main subject of previous portions of this book. This type of immunity is designated *innate immunity*, and it is found in many primitive organisms such as insects and other invertebrates. What is particularly remarkable is that the ancient immune system still exists in humans and other higher organisms and that it interacts with and guides modern immune responses. How innate immunity and the closely related phenomenon of inflammation contribute both to protective immunity and to a variety of diseases such as colitis, metabolic diseases, and cancer is also the subject of this section.

Part six considers the role of the immune system in HIV infection and in causing inflammatory diseases, including allergic diseases, as well as how it can be used to treat cancer and how it must be controlled to allow tissue and organ transplantation. It includes the story of a family tragedy that emphasizes the need to have better tools both for the immune system's fight against cancer and for the control of the immune system to make bone marrow transplantation an even more effective lifesaving therapy.

The book closes with a conclusion, in which I consider the future of the field, and an epilogue, where I argue forcefully that generous support of research in immunological science and the other branches of medicine (support that was present in previous years) could yield unprecedented future dividends in terms of advances in prevention and treatment of disease.

In this era of newly emerging diseases, such as Ebola, understanding how the immune system works and the nature of its protection is more important than ever.

I | IMMUNOLOGY

1

Defense and Danger

The immune system has immense power to protect us from the ravages of infection through its ability to kill disease-causing microbes or to eliminate them from the body. But the power of the immune system is a double-edged sword. Its power to destroy infectious agents, if it goes wrong, can have devastating effects on the body—resulting sometimes in life-threatening diseases. In this first chapter, I illustrate the power of the immune system to protect us, as exemplified by the eradication of smallpox, and the danger the immune system poses, shown by one of the many diseases in which immune cells destroy normal tissue, in this case type 1 diabetes, caused by the immune destruction of insulin-producing cells. Finally, I demonstrate the consequences of a crippled immune system, by describing the ravages of HIV infection and the susceptibility to infection seen in AIDS and other immunodeficiency diseases.

Farewell (and Good Riddance) to Smallpox

On May 8, 1980, in Geneva, Switzerland, the World Health Assembly accepted the report of the Global Commission for the Certification of Smallpox Eradication that smallpox had been eliminated from the planet. This was an accomplishment of stunning magnitude. Almost certainly, it was the first time that a lethal microbe had been eradicated from the world through a concerted public health effort.

The commission's report was based on its finding that Ali Maow Maalin, a cook at the hospital in Merca, Somalia, was the last person to be naturally infected with the virus that causes smallpox. He contracted the infection on October 26, 1977, but did not transmit the virus to anyone else. Despite intense surveillance, no naturally transmitted infections were detected between Maalin's diagnosis and the May 8, 1980, announcement. Indeed, to our knowledge, no non-laboratory-transmitted smallpox infections have occurred since then.

The significance of smallpox eradication cannot be overemphasized. Variola, the virus that causes smallpox, afflicted humans for millennia. Smallpox has probably been responsible for more deaths than any other infectious agent, possibly more than any other medical condition.

The Americas were free of smallpox before the arrival of Europeans. The virus arrived with the newcomers and devastated native populations, as none among them was immune. It is likely that the relative ease with which a small number of Spaniards subjugated much of North and South America was materially aided by the disruption of ordered native society due to the vast number of deaths from smallpox and other infectious agents new to the Americas.

Efforts to prevent smallpox were made in many countries throughout history, usually involving the exposure of an individual to what was thought to be a weak form of the disease-causing agent (this was long before the discovery of viruses). The hope was that the treated person would contract a mild illness and obtain the lifelong resistance that occurred in those who recovered from a natural smallpox infection. It was Edward Jenner's introduction of vaccination, in 1796 in Gloucestershire, England, that transformed this haphazard and dangerous effort into one that was highly effective and safe, leading the way to all subsequent vaccines.[1] Although Jenner's work was done almost a century before the development of immunology as a science, in many respects, it represents the field's greatest achievement.

Jenner knew that milkmaids often became ill with cowpox, which caused a mild infection. Once they had recovered, they rarely contracted smallpox. Today, we know that the virus responsible for cowpox is vaccinia, a close relative of variola. Jenner reasoned that intentionally infecting individuals with the cowpox agent might protect them against smallpox infection and, if successful, could provide to the population at large the resistance to smallpox of previously cowpox-infected milkmaids.

In 1796, Jenner extracted fluid from pustules on the skin of Sarah Nelmes, who had a natural cowpox infection. He injected this fluid into the skin of James Phipps. After Phipps recovered from the mild illness caused by the cowpox virus, Jenner intentionally inoculated him with fluid from pustules of a patient with authentic smallpox. Although such treatment would have been expected to transmit smallpox, Phipps did not develop signs of infection, implying that inoculation with cowpox virus had protected him against smallpox.

Jenner's experiment violates modern norms of medical research. Intentionally infecting a person with the smallpox virus would surely be unacceptable today. However, in his era, it was common practice for doctors to introduce extracts from pustules of individuals with mild cases of smallpox into children and adults in an effort to prevent a natural, and presumably much more virulent, infection. This practice, *variolation* (derived from variola), was dangerous because some of those inoculated developed severe cases of smallpox and died.[2] But fear of smallpox was so great that, though controversial, variolation was often carried out, so Jenner's methodology may not have seemed out of line at the time.[3]

Even after the efficacy of administration of vaccinia (hence *vaccination*) had been established, some rejected its use, a view echoed today by those opposed to any vaccination. Despite the opposition, use of the vaccine was rapidly taken up and the incidence of smallpox in western European countries declined markedly by 1820, although epidemics continued to occur due to a poorly appreciated waning of immunity and the need for revaccination. The UK Vaccination Act of 1853 required that every child whose health permitted be vaccinated within three or four months of birth.

The smallpox virus cannot survive outside of a host, and it has no hosts other than humans. The disease is an acute one in which the virus is either eradicated by the infected individual or the infected person dies. If a sufficiently large number of people in any population are vaccinated, and thus are resistant to infection, the virus will disappear from that group since it will find no new hosts to infect. This phenomenon is often referred to by the term *herd immunity*. Basically, if a large proportion of a group of people is resistant to infection, the infectious agent will die out because the likelihood that it will find a susceptible individual before it loses infectivity will fall below a critical number and thus, within a predictable length of time, no new infections will occur. Based on these considerations, it seemed very likely that smallpox could be eliminated if all populations were so protected.

Acting on this knowledge, the World Health Organization launched the Intensified Smallpox Eradication Programme in 1967 with the goal of global elimination within ten years. The eradication campaign utilized an intensive program of vaccination in locations where the virus was still being transmitted, using strategies aimed at preventing the virus from spreading from infected individuals to new hosts. When a case was detected, everyone who may have had contact with the infected individual, be they family members or casual contacts, immediately received the vaccine if they had not been vaccinated already. This approach was termed *ring vaccination*. Dr. Donald A. Henderson, later dean of the Johns Hopkins School of Public Health, led the campaign to eradicate smallpox. He and his team achieved success just ahead of schedule. The chain of viral transmission was interrupted and the virus was eliminated from nature.

Smallpox virus continued to be maintained in many laboratories throughout the world, but when a laboratory accident in Birmingham, United Kingdom, in 1978, resulted in a limited outbreak and one death, the World Health Organization proposed that the virus be maintained in only two locations: the Centers for Disease Control and Prevention (CDC) in Atlanta, Georgia, and the VECTOR Institute in Koltisovo in the USSR.

Discussions about whether these stocks of the virus should be destroyed have gone on since then. The argument for destroying the virus was that it would ensure that it could not be accidently (or intentionally) reintroduced. However, others reasoned that without any samples of the virus, it would not be possible to find better treatments or better vaccines in case smallpox was reintroduced somehow. This concern has some merit, as stocks of virus might still exist. In the summer of 2014, vials of the smallpox virus were discovered in a laboratory of the Food and Drug Administration in Bethesda, Maryland. They appear to have dated from the 1950s and obviously had been forgotten. After testing, the virus was destroyed. But it would not be surprising if long forgotten variola stocks hide in other laboratories throughout the world.

Even more concerning is the possibility that terrorist groups and others may have obtained smallpox cultures with the intention of developing a bioterror weapon. With the cessation of smallpox vaccination, the majority of most populations are susceptible to infection. In the United States, compulsory smallpox vaccination ended in 1972, so essentially everyone born after that date is susceptible and probably many in the older group are as well since the protection offered by vaccination wanes with time.

It has been suggested that variola could be made even more lethal for use as a bioterror weapon by introducing new genes into it that would make the virus more deadly than the natural agent. One way would be to produce a virus that had the capacity to impair the ability of the infected individual to develop a protective immune response. This is more than an academic possibility. It has been done for a virus that is a close relative of smallpox virus. That virus, ectromelia, causes mousepox, which has high lethality for mice. Scientists in Canberra, Australia, and in St. Louis, Missouri, engineered the mousepox virus to express the gene for interleukin-4 (IL-4). IL-4 is a cytokine, a small protein made by white blood cells that targets other cells and changes their behavior in important ways. My colleagues and I discovered IL-4 in the early 1980s. One of its functions is to redirect the immune response so that it is less effective against certain types of infectious agents and more effective against parasites. The IL-4-engineered ectromelia was more lethal than the natural virus and would cause death even in mice that had been vaccinated and were immune to "normal" ectromelia. Whether terrorist groups would carry out such a genetic engineering effort is speculative, but the concern certainly exists.

The eradication of smallpox naturally raised the question as to whether other infectious agents could be eliminated. The cattle viral disease rinderpest (German for "cattle plague"), which is highly lethal and has been a particular scourge in Africa, has recently been eliminated by aggressive vaccination of at-risk cattle. On May 25, 2011, the World Organisation for Animal Health announced that all countries were now free of rinderpest.

Both polio and measles could, in principle, be eliminated. For both diseases, there are highly effective vaccines; in both cases, humans are the only host; and the diagnosis of the infection can be made with certainty so that the status of a population can be accurately determined. If these viruses were eliminated from humans, the virus could no longer sustain itself in nature.

The World Health Organization has made the eradication of polio a priority. Mass vaccination has already eliminated the disease from the Western Hemisphere, the last naturally transmitted case occurring in Peru in 1991. Europe, too, has been certified as polio-free. Indeed, India, until recently a country in which the virus was being transmitted (an endemic country), was reported polio-free in 2012. In 2014, however, polio was still endemic in Pakistan, Afghanistan, and Nigeria, and cases were reported in

Somalia, Equatorial Guinea, Iraq, Cameroon, Syria, and Ethiopia. Perhaps more worrisome was that polio virus was shown to be present in sewage in Cairo and in Israel.[4]

The principle of vaccination has now been widely applied. Vaccines originally were weakened (attenuated) forms of a virus or bacterium that caused a disease, but more recently, effective vaccines have been based on protein or polysaccharide components of the disease-causing agents. The US Food and Drug Administration has approved almost fifty vaccines for human use, and many more are now under development. The CDC recommends that healthy infants and children receive vaccinations on at least six different doctor visits. As many as six vaccines may be given at a single visit to the pediatrician.

Vaccines have probably had a greater impact on human health than any other human intervention, with the possible exception of modern practices of sanitation. But great challenges still need to be met. Effective vaccines for the three greatest infectious killers of humans, the AIDS virus, HIV; *M. tuberculosis*, the bacterium that causes tuberculosis; and the plasmodia, the organisms that cause malaria, still remain to be developed, although much effort has been made and continues to be made to develop vaccines for each of these pathogens.

How the Immune System Causes Diabetes

A counterpoint to the great accomplishment of the eradication of smallpox through the mobilization of the immune system by vaccination is the impact of immune responses "gone wrong." This situation can be illustrated by an event played out all too often. A young girl is brought by her parents to a hospital emergency room. She is in a coma, after having had severe abdominal pains and nausea and vomiting. She has a strong smell of acetone on her breath. The emergency room doctors quickly recognize that the child has ketoacidosis, a severe condition stemming from metabolic abnormalities that occur in the absence of insulin. Without insulin, the body uses fat rather than glucose as a source of energy. "Burning" fat for energy results in the excess production of "ketone bodies," including acetone, which acidify the blood, resulting in the ketoacidosis in this severely ill young child.

The girl's doctors promptly treat her with intravenous fluids, sodium and potassium replenishment, and administration of insulin, controlling this life-threatening situation. She and her parents are told that she has type 1 diabetes mellitus (also known as juvenile diabetes or insulin-dependent diabetes mellitus).

The immune response that had been so beneficial in eliminating small-pox has revealed an entirely different, and very dangerous, face. Cells of the immune system, some of which are known as killer T cells, destroyed the insulin-producing cells of this child's pancreas. Her T cells had recognized the β cells of her islets of Langerhans, the insulin-producing cells in her pancreas, and had developed into killers that targeted these cells and destroyed them. By the time her diabetes was apparent, these killer T cells had destroyed the great majority of the child's β cells so that she was unable to produce sufficient insulin to metabolize glucose properly.

Normally, the tissues of an individual should not be targets of immune responses; several processes, collectively referred to as *immunologic tolerance*, prevent such self-reactivity by eliminating or suppressing potentially self-reactive cells. When this child's killer T cells attacked her own β cells, a key group of cells were destroyed in a process referred to as *autoimmunity*.

Children develop diabetic coma every day. The number of new cases of type 1 diabetes in the United States has been estimated as ten per hundred thousand persons per year, a frequency similar to that of much of the western world. In Finland, which has the world's highest incidence, there are forty-five new cases per hundred thousand each year. Type 1 diabetes is believed to be on the rise in many countries, including the United States. That means there are approximately eighty-six cases of type 1 diabetes diagnosed in the United States each day. About one quarter of these new cases are in children whose disease has progressed to the point that they are in a diabetic coma at the time of diagnosis.

Unfortunately, attacks of the cells of the immune system on self-tissues and organs are all too common. Among the other diseases that result from such autoimmune attack are rheumatoid arthritis, systemic lupus erythematosus (SLE), multiple sclerosis, inflammatory bowel diseases (ulcerative colitis and Crohn's disease), thyroiditis, myasthenia gravis, and psoriasis. Many of these autoimmune diseases, particularly SLE, are far more common in women than in men.

The damage that the immune system may cause is even greater than that indicated by this impressive set of diseases. The immune response and its attendant inflammatory processes play a major role in the cause and progression of arteriosclerosis and its complications of heart attack and stroke and may contribute to the more common form of diabetes, type 2, as well as to development of nonalcoholic fatty liver and its complications, liver cirrhosis and some forms of liver cancer.

New treatments and, more importantly, preventatives for these immune or inflammatory disorders are desperately needed. One of the most hopeful signs is that the inflammation that is key to the progression of rheumatoid arthritis and Crohn's disease can be markedly reduced by the administration of drugs that block the action of a key substance that causes inflammation, the cytokine *tumor necrosis factor alpha* (TNFα). Treatment with TNFα inhibitors has helped markedly in the treatment of rheumatoid arthritis.[5] Blocking other inflammatory mediators appears to have a similar effect. An antibody that blocks the action of another cytokine, interleukin-6, is also very effective in the treatment of rheumatoid arthritis. Antibodies to different cytokines are effective in treating psoriasis.

Recently, patients suffering from a set of genetically determined auto-inflammatory diseases have been shown to make remarkable recoveries when treated with an inhibitor of interleukin-1 (IL-1), yet another cytokine important in mediating inflammatory and immune responses. These diseases are due to excess production of this pro-inflammatory cytokine or enhanced sensitivity to the cytokine. We need to improve on the currently available treatments and to extend them more generally.

A New, Terrifying Infection

Both vaccine-mediated smallpox eradication and the destruction of the insulin-producing cells of the pancreas by killer T cells represent the power of the immune response, one to promote health, the other to degrade it. A third possibility is the immune system failing to carry out its functions, in which case the outcome can be devastating. Human immunodeficiency virus (HIV) infection and the attendant acquired immunodeficiency syndrome (AIDS) burst into our consciousness in 1980. In many places, but particularly in New York City, Los Angeles, San Francisco, and Paris, young gay men acquired HIV as a result of unprotected sex with an infected partner. Both these young men and their sexual partners were unaware of their infection. Over the next several weeks, the newly HIV-infected men probably developed the flulike symptoms of an acute viral infection, but then, at least initially, they seemed well. It is likely that they went on to have unprotected sex with others and that, quite unknowingly, they transmitted the virus to these new partners, propagating the nascent epidemic.

In 1980 and 1981, patients with a very unusual pneumonia, caused by the unicellular fungus *Pneumocystis carinii*,[6] began to appear in doctors' offices and emergency rooms in substantial numbers. Previously, pneumocystis pneumonia had been a relatively rare infection, observed mainly in people with profoundly suppressed immune systems, particularly those being treated with potent anticancer drugs. However, these patients were generally young men with no history of taking immunosuppressive drugs.

At the same time, large numbers of individuals were developing what had been a rare skin cancer, Kaposi's sarcoma, which usually presents as extensive purplish skin lesions. Kaposi's sarcoma generally had been confined to older men, particularly of Eastern European and Mediterranean heritage. These new cases of Kaposi's sarcoma were occurring in precisely the same group that was developing pneumocystis pneumonia, young gay men in large metropolitan areas.

In 1981, the condition underlying both the susceptibility to pneumocystis pneumonia and other opportunistic infections and the development of Kaposi's sarcoma was recognized as a new entity. Several names were initially proposed, but AIDS (SIDA in France) became the accepted nomenclature.

Luc Montagnier and Françoise Barre-Sinoussi at the Institut Pasteur isolated a virus from a lymph node biopsy of a patient in 1983 at the Hôpital Bichat in Paris. That virus proved to be the causative agent of AIDS. Montagnier and Barre-Sinoussi received the 2008 Nobel Prize in Physiology or Medicine for this discovery. Montagnier first named the virus *lymphadenopathy-associated virus*, since the patient from whom the virus had been isolated had an acute infection associated with enlarged lymph nodes. Later, the virus was called HIV.

HIV was independently isolated at the National Institutes of Health (NIH) in Bethesda, Maryland, in 1984 by a research group led by Robert Gallo. Gallo and his colleagues developed an effective blood test for HIV infection that both strengthened the argument that this virus was truly the cause of AIDS and allowed earlier diagnosis. The development of the blood test was a key step forward because it allowed blood bankers to test each unit of blood to determine whether it contained HIV. Because of this advance, the safety of the blood supply was assured.

The first verifiable instance of HIV infection appears to date to 1959, based on the study of stored blood samples in Kinshasa, now in the Democratic Republic of Congo.[7] A detailed analysis of the genes of this virus and of a virus isolated slightly later led to the estimate that HIV was being transmitted among humans since the 1930s or even earlier.

HIV developed as a result of a rare transmission of a chimpanzee virus, known as simian immunodeficiency virus–chimpanzee, into humans and the adaptation of that virus so that it could be transmitted from human to human. However, it was only in the late 1970s and early 1980s that HIV began to rapidly infect large numbers of individuals whose behaviors put them at high risk of infection. As of 2014, UNAIDS, the international body with the responsibility to track the disease, estimates that about 34 million people are infected with HIV and that the infection causes approximately 1.7 million deaths each year.

HIV infection illustrates the consequence of the lack of or diminished function of the immune system. The immune system protects us against becoming infected with the large number of potentially pathogenic microbes with which we share our living space. HIV places us at risk of infection with these microbes largely because it results in the loss of key cells of the immune system, the CD4 T cells. In the weeks immediately after HIV infection, there is a remarkable loss of CD4 T cells from the gastrointestinal tract and other mucosal tissues. While the mechanisms resulting in progression of HIV-infected individuals to AIDS are complex and still the subject of debate, the early loss of the majority of gastrointestinal T cells appears to be a critical step in this process.

Patients with advanced HIV infection have greatly increased susceptibility to microorganisms that pose little or no threat to healthy adults. Infections with these organisms are referred to as *opportunistic*. Pneumocystis pneumonia is an example of an opportunistic infection.

HIV infection and AIDS illustrate how central a functioning immune system is to our survival. Another example that brings home the importance of immunity is the great susceptibility to infection of children born with major defects in their immune system such as those with *severe combined immunodeficiency* (SCID). Children with SCID will not survive unless they receive a bone marrow transplant from a normal donor. David Vetter, born with this disease in 1971, was kept in a clean "bubble," in which he was protected from the outside environment, where he survived until 1984. The plight of people who have SCID highlights the essential role of the immune system in the fight against microbial pathogens.

Whether viewed from its capacity to defend (as in the case of the smallpox vaccination) or to endanger (as with the onset of type 1 diabetes), the immune system affects aspects of health we often take for granted. The importance of the immune system for resistance to the great array of microbes we encounter each day is shown by the heightened susceptibility of people who have AIDS or other immunodeficiencies to infection with agents that most of us control with no difficulty. In the next chapter, we take a closer look at the precise path of an immune response by examining one of the more surprising outbreaks of the late twentieth century.

2

Tracing an Immune Response

In 1976, more than two hundred of the attendees at the American Legion Convention in Philadelphia, honoring the two hundredth anniversary of the Declaration of Independence, became severely ill from a previously unknown respiratory infection. Thirty-four died. All of the affected individuals had stayed at the Bellevue-Stratford Hotel. After much investigation, the cause of their illness was shown to be a bacteria not previously known to infect humans. The microorganism, *Legionella pneumophila*, and the disease, Legionnaires' disease, were named to memorialize the victims.

Legionella was found growing in the cooling tower of the hotel's air conditioning system. This discovery prompted new regulations for these systems. Possibly in response to the great concern raised by the outbreak, the Bellevue-Stratford Hotel was sold, the guest rooms completely gutted and renovated, and the hotel reopened with a new name.

When a *pathogen*, a disease-causing microbe such as legionella, enters the body, various aspects of the immune response are brought to bear as the body struggles to control that pathogen. Let's trace the events that occur when the immune system mounts a defense against infection.

Physical Barriers

Legionella is aspirated in droplets and infects cells lining the air sacs of the lungs (*epithelial cells*) and cells that are specialized to ingest foreign materials that are found within the lung air sacs (*macrophages*).

The body's first strategy in resisting infection with legionella, or other potential attackers, is to prevent the bacteria from gaining access to the cells it can infect. It achieves this by erecting a physical barrier. For the lung, that barrier is the action of specialized cells lining the upper airway. These cells have hairlike structures (*cilia*) on the surfaces that face the interior of the airway. The cilia beat in a coordinated manner toward the mouth. Also, the airway is lined by a layer of mucus that traps entering microorganisms. Trapped bacteria are swept upward and out by this mucociliary escalator and are either swallowed and destroyed by stomach acid or are spit out.

This upper airway barrier may be damaged by smoking, by chronic asthma and chronic bronchitis, and by certain viral infections. Individuals with damaged barriers are more susceptible to infections of the bronchi and lung. But in healthy individuals, the mucociliary mechanism is a powerful means to maintain sterility in the lower airways and the lung.

Innate Immunity

For many of the attendees at the American Legion convention, the physical barrier was not sufficient to keep legionella from penetrating to the lower portions of the airway. In these instances, a form of immunity known as *innate immunity* swung into action. Evolutionarily, innate immunity is ancient. It differs from *adaptive immunity* in that it is not based on antibodies or the other type of responses that occur when we are vaccinated, the expansion and action of T cells. Rather, innate immunity represents a built-in response that depends on the capacity of highly conserved molecules to recognize certain important microbial factors.

Once legionella organisms have gained entrance to the lower airway but have not yet entered a cell, several types of immune system cells can detect them. These cells are principally macrophages and lung-tissue cells that have elements on their surfaces called toll-like receptors (TLRs). TLRs and related molecules can recognize components of legionella. This recognition event causes a chain of biochemical responses within cells that leads to the production of key molecules, *cytokines*, that can act on many other cells to make them more resistant to infection or help them destroy the legionella that enter them. These cytokines, prominent among them interleukin-1 (IL-1), not only mobilize cells of the innate immune system to help destroy the legionella, but they are also responsible for many of the symptoms felt by the infected individual. IL-1 can act on specialized cells in the brain that regulate body temperature and lead to the fever and chills that occur with infections like Legionnaires' disease.

Those legionella organisms that do find their way into the interior of the lung cells that line the airway encounter a new set of innate immune recognition elements. The detection of legionella components by these innate recognition elements within the cell signals the cell to make more IL-1 and other cytokines, also mobilizing cells of the innate immune system. In particular, IL-1 recruits a type of white blood cell known as the *neutrophil*. Neutrophils are produced in the bone marrow and can be found circulating in the blood. When neutrophils detect IL-1 produced in the airway, they flood into the lung and will be drawn directly to the site of the infection.

Amazingly, these rapidly recruited neutrophils "know" where to go. They do so because the infection stimulates the production of yet another set of molecules of the immune system that attract cells to a particular site. These molecules, called *chemokines*, are secreted from the site of infection. The incoming neutrophils bind the chemokine, resulting in a biochemical signal inside the neutrophil. This signal impels the neutrophils to follow the gradient of the chemokine toward its source, ensuring that large numbers of neutrophils arrive at the site of infection.

Neutrophils have many mechanisms through which they can help to clear infections. First, they are good at ingesting the microorganisms and killing them. They also make and secrete many substances that can directly destroy the bacteria. A very recently discovered and quite remarkable defense function of neutrophils is *netosis*. Netosis is triggered by the death of the incoming neutrophils. The dying neutrophils release neutrophil extracellular traps (NETs) consisting of contents of the cells' nuclei that are protein structures coated with antibacterial elements. Bacteria are caught and killed in these NETs.

The intracellular recognition of the legionella also causes the cell to make cytokines called *interferons*. Interferons endow the infected cell with several mechanisms through which it can control and destroy the infecting organism.

All of these events occur very rapidly and can, in some cases, completely rid the body of the infection. In other cases, the innate immune system acts to diminish the effective numbers of the infecting pathogen and slow the rate at which the pathogen can expand so that there is sufficient time for the adaptive immune system to swing into action.

Adaptive Immunity

The mobilization and activation of the cells of the innate immune system in the lung in response to the entry of legionella occurs in parallel with a slower, but in the end highly effective, response. White blood cells of a special type, *lymphocytes*, undergo massive expansion. Some of these lymphocytes (and their descendants) produce antibodies to legionella; others, the T cells, mediate various bacterial control mechanisms.

In the lung, in addition to the macrophages and the epithelial cells, which are the principal cells infected and the cells in which the recognition events that mobilize the innate immune system occur, there is a population of highly specialized cells, *dendritic cells*. Until a microorganism appears, dendritic cells are in a quiescent state. With the appearance of the legionella bacteria, the dendritic cells become activated as a result of both their own recognition mechanisms and their response to signals from the infected cells.

Once activated, the dendritic cells in the lung take up intact legionella bacteria and bacterial fragments. The dendritic cells now become highly mobile and capable of responding to chemokines made in the lymph nodes that drain the lung. Following the gradient of these chemokines, the activated dendritic cells carry their ingested load of legionella and legionella fragments from the lung, through the lymphatic vessels, to the tracheobronchial lymph nodes that drain the lung tissue.

As these dendritic cells migrate from the lung to the lymph node, they activate a specialized metabolic program through which they break down the legionella proteins into small fragments. A set of highly specialized molecules designated *major histocompatibility complex* (MHC) molecules then carry these fragments to the surface of the dendritic cells. The legionella fragments bound to MHC molecules will be recognized in the lymph node by a specific set of T lymphocytes, those that have cell surface receptors that can bind the complex of legionella fragments and MHC molecules on the surface of the dendritic cell.

This process represents a critical difference between the innate and adaptive immune systems. In the innate immune system, all the cells of the same type have the same capacity to recognize and respond to legionella. But this is not true of the key cells of the adaptive immune system, the lymphocytes. Lymphocytes differ from one another in terms of what they can recognize. Each lymphocyte has a different antigen-recognition receptor, and any antigen can only be recognized by a very few lymphocytes. Thus, the legionella protein fragments will only be detected by a small minority of the T lymphocytes in the lymph node. The frequency of "legionella-specific" T lymphocytes may be one in a hundred thousand, or even less. But once those specific lymphocytes recognize the legionella fragment, they receive a powerful stimulation that results in very rapid cell division. In less than a week, the responding T cells may increase in number ten thousand times, creating an enormous population of T cells specific for legionella.

As the T cells expand in the lymph node, they undergo a striking change. The previously small, resting lymphocytes acquire new properties through which they can directly or indirectly destroy or control the legionella. Among these new properties are production of the cytokine *interferon-gamma* (IFNγ), which equips the infected cells to destroy the legionella; acquisition of the capacity of the T cells themselves to kill the legionella-infected cells; and development of the ability to aid another lymphocyte type, the B cells, to make antibodies that block legionella's capacity to infect new cells or that mobilize inflammatory mechanisms to destroy the legionella bacteria.

Of course, simply having the capacity to control legionella would be of little value if the T cells remained in the draining lymph node, as the legionella infection is in the lung, not the lymph node. Accordingly, the now-expanded number of legionella-specific T cells leave the lymph node and travel to the site of the infection where they mediate the functions that control legionella. They also can migrate to other lymph nodes and to the spleen so that they equip the body for future responses.

If all goes well, the legionella organisms will be completely eliminated and the infection terminated. Indeed, legionella only causes severe consequences in those whose immune responses are impaired, either because their physical barriers to block entry are impaired, their innate responses are inadequate, or they have defects in their adaptive responses. In these individuals, the race between the bacterium and the response goes to the pathogen, and the consequences can be severe, including death.

In the more favorable outcomes, once the legionella are eliminated, the damage caused by the infection and by the cells responding to the infection must be repaired. This repair process takes some time, but the lungs of the infected individual then return to normal.

In the patient who has recovered from a legionella infection, the innate immune system will gradually lose its activated state and return to a condition much as it was before infection. It would still be capable of limiting the growth of newly introduced legionella organisms but not, in a major way, any differently from how it responded to its first encounter with legionella.

By contrast, the adaptive immune system displays *immunologic memory*. It will respond very differently to a second encounter with legionella. While many of the legionella-specific lymphocytes that expanded in response to being stimulated by the legionella antigens will die, some of these cells will survive and be available, as memory cells, in much larger numbers than existed prior to the infection. If a new legionella infection occurs, the response mounted will be much more rapid and much larger in magnitude. Furthermore, because the lymphocytes are mobile, the memory cells will be distributed throughout the body so that a legionella infection introduced through another site can be dealt with effectively.

Equally important, the antibodies that were produced in response to the first legionella infection will persist for long periods. These antibodies can often entirely prevent new legionella organisms from gaining access to the cells of the lung and completely block a new infection. Such antibodies provide the individual with *sterilizing immunity*.

The immune responses to a legionella invasion also occur with other types of infections, those due to extracellular bacteria, viruses, and parasites, and those in other parts of the body such as the gastrointestinal tract, the skin, or the genitourinary tract. These responses are similar in principle but not in detail. Virtually every microorganism is unique and occupies its own niche within the body. The immune response mounted against each is also unique, following common principles but adapting them so that the response is well suited to the threat. Researchers and scientists designing new vaccines keep foremost in their minds both the details of how the microorganism causes disease and the character of the immune response best suited to control the microorganism.

The body's response to an antigen threat such as legionella is thus complex and involves the overlapping innate and adaptive immune systems. These systems, working in a coordinated manner, provide an extremely powerful protection against the vast array of potentially disease-causing microbes.

3

The Laws of Immunology

Universality, Tolerance, and Appropriateness

To combat an infection such as legionella, the immune system, in both its innate and adaptive aspects, mounts a coordinated response to identify and destroy the pathogen. The response needs to be tailored to the type of infection, with legionella representing one of many distinct types of threats. But what overarching rules govern the responses of the immune system? Three principles inform the behavior of the cells and products of the immune system. I prefer to refer to them as the laws of immunity: universality, tolerance, and appropriateness. But to appreciate these laws, we first need to understand the central information-carrying cells of the immune system, the lymphocytes.

Lymphocytes

Lymphocytes are the cells that make the specific responses to pathogens. Other cells within the immune system interact with and control or modulate the function of the lymphocytes, but it is the lymphocytes that call the tune. Lymphocytes are small white blood cells that, in their resting state, are basically nuclei with a small rim of cytoplasm (figure 3.1). They are found in large numbers in the lymph nodes, spleen, tonsils, and the organized lymphoid tissue of the intestinal tract, as well as in the bone marrow and the thymus. But lymphocytes occur in virtually all tissues and organs of the body, usually in relatively small numbers. Large numbers of lymphocytes will enter the site of a local infection.

Our knowledge of the centrality of the lymphocyte in the immune response is relatively recent. When I was in medical school, we were taught immunology as part of a course in medical microbiology, the science of in-

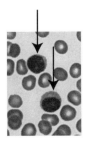

Figure 3.1. Lymphocytes (indicated by arrows) are the information-carrying cells of the immune system. (Courtesy of Dr. Kristine Krafts, Department of Pathology, University of Minnesota School of Medicine)

fectious agents. My professor of microbiology, who had been the president of the American Association of Immunologists, was deeply skeptical about the function of lymphocytes. Even a few years earlier, most scientists had no conception of what lymphocytes did. Lymphocytes are so unprepossessing in appearance that many believed their chief function was to serve as nutrients for cells that were thought to be more important in antimicrobial responses, such as macrophages, the cells that "eat" bacteria through a process called *phagocytosis*.

It was not until the 1950s and early 1960s that scientists understood how essential lymphocytes were to mounting immune responses. In a series of brilliant experiments, James Gowans and his colleagues at Oxford University showed that small lymphocytes in the rat (such as those in figure 3.1) continuously circulate through the blood and the lymph. To demonstrate the importance of lymphocytes in immune responses, Gowans asked what would happen to an animal's ability to make an immune response if these cells were removed. He knew that the lymph fluid was highly enriched in lymphocytes and that almost all of the lymph in the body, moving through vessels called lymphatics, flows into the thoracic duct, the largest lymphatic. The contents of the thoracic duct enter the blood system through the vena cava, the great vein that enters the right side of the heart.

Gowans inserted a small tube into the thoracic duct of a rat and drained the fluid from the duct for twenty-four hours. Drainage over this period of time caused a marked diminution in the total number of lymphocytes in the spleen and lymph nodes and resulted in a striking fall in the rat's capacity to make an antibody response when immunized with a test antigen. This was strong evidence that lymphocytes were important in mounting antibody responses.

Gowans's work showed that lymphocytes were needed to make antibody responses, but it did not prove that lymphocytes carried the specificity of the immune response. Another researcher, Avrion Mitchison, had just earned his PhD at Oxford University, under the supervision of another great figure of English immunology, Peter Medawar. Mitchison reasoned that by taking lymphocytes from an animal immunized with some particular antigen and injecting those lymphocytes into another similar, but unimmunized, animal, he could test whether the transferred lymphocytes endowed the recipient with the immunity of the donor. To do the lymphocyte transfer experiments necessary to test whether the lymphocytes were the specific cells of the immune system, he realized he had to use inbred mice, mice that are genetically identical to one another. This would be necessary to avoid the rejection that occurs when cells from one individual are transferred to another individual that is genetically different.

Inbred mice were first developed by Clarence Little, then a young scientist at Harvard. Little realized that by a program of interbreeding many successive generations of brother and sister mice from an initial cross, he could obtain animals that were essentially genetically identical and that were homozygous (had the same "version," or *allele*, of a gene) at every site in the genome. He began his derivation of the first inbred mouse strain in 1909. After serving in the US Army in World War I, he returned to this effort. Recognized for his overall brilliance, he was appointed president of the University of Maine in 1922, at the age of thirty-three; three years later, he moved to the University of Michigan. With support he obtained from donors in the automobile industry, particularly the Jackson family of the Hudson Motor Car Company and the Ford family, he established a dedicated center for the development and study of inbred strains of mice in Bar Harbor, Maine. Currently, there are more than 5,000 strains of inbred mice maintained at the Jackson Laboratory, which is the leading source of inbred laboratory mice for scientists throughout the world.

Mitchison came to Bar Harbor to do his postdoctoral work. He used techniques he had learned from Medawar and the unrivaled mouse genetic resources of the Jackson Laboratory to carry out his key experiment. He implanted cells from a tumor that had arisen in a particular mouse strain into other mice of the same strain and waited until the mice had rejected the tumors. He showed this was an immunologically specific event since these mice would rapidly reject a second inoculation of the same tumor cells but would only slowly reject tumor cells of a different type. He then took lymphocytes from the spleens and lymph nodes of mice that had rejected a particular tumor and injected them intravenously into other mice of the same inbred strain and tested the recipients to see if they had acquired the immunity of the donor. The striking result was that the recipients gained the capacity to immediately reject the tumor against which the donor had been immunized but not other tumors. Mitchison's experiment established not only that lymphocytes were important in making immune responses but that they carried the information that specified which antigens an animal had been immunized against.[1]

B Lymphocytes and T Lymphocytes

Immune responses can manifest themselves in several ways. Antibodies are critical for protection against the bacteria that cause pneumococcal pneumonia and many other similar bacteria, particularly those that grow in the bodily fluids that are outside of cells.

There is, however, another important type of immune response, *cellular immunity*, that does not involve antibodies. Cellular immunity is crucial in protecting against tuberculosis and other bacterial infections in which the bacteria grow within cells. It was only in the late 1960s that it was appreciated that these two forms of immunity could be mapped to two distinct types of lymphocytes. The cells that develop into antibody-producing cells are designated B lymphocytes, whereas those responsible for mediating cellular immunity are designated T lymphocytes. B and T lymphocytes are different from one another in their origin, in the key molecules they express, and in their functions.

The designation *T lymphocyte* was based on the finding, particularly by Jacques Miller and Graham Mitchell at the Walter and Eliza Hall Institute of Medical Research in Melbourne, that these cells undergo critical steps in their development within the thymus. For this reason, these cells were initially termed *thymus-derived lymphocytes*, but over the years the simpler name T lymphocytes has come to dominate. The cells that actually develop into antibody-producing cells do not differentiate in the thymus. They are derived directly from cells in the bone marrow. Precursors of antibody-producing cells were often designated *bone marrow–derived lymphocytes*, but the term *B lymphocytes* is now in general use.

The separation of antibody-based immune responses and cellular immunity and the intimation that the first is solely due to the action of B lymphocytes and the second to T lymphocytes represents an oversimplification. Although B lymphocytes, when appropriately stimulated, develop into antibody-producing cells, they often require the action of T cells in order to undergo this development. For this reason, the set of T lymphocytes that help the B cells develop into antibody-producing cells are referred to as *helper T cells*, or *Th cells*.[2]

While I was on a short fellowship in Mitchison's laboratory in London, Mitchison showed me some experiments he had done in which he had immunized mice with a chemical conjugate of a protein and a small organic molecule (a hapten, more on which in chapter 6). For simplicity, I'll call the protein X. He also immunized other mice with another protein alone; I'll call it Y. He then transferred cells from both the hapten-X- and the Y-immunized mice to inbred mice of the same strain and found that they would make anti-hapten antibody if challenged with hapten conjugated to protein Y. Thus, although the mice had never been immunized with hapten-Y, they acquired responsiveness to this conjugate by having been separately immunized with Y alone, implying that specific cells could participate in recognizing the hapten-Y conjugate. By the same reasoning the hapten-X immunization endowed some cells in that animal with the ability to recognize the hapten even though it was part of a different conjugate, implying that there were hapten-specific cells. What he later showed was that the hapten-specific cells were B cells and the carrier specific cells were T cells, providing a very elegant demonstration of the cooperation between helper T cells and B cells.

Selection versus Instruction

One of the great debates during the development of immunology was how specificity is achieved, that is, how the immune system is able to appropriately target specific pathogens. The initial controversy centered on whether the information necessary to mount a response against a foreign substance preexisted in the individual and the foreign antigenic substance selected the response from a preexisting menu or whether the system was essentially a blank slate and the antigen "taught" the immune system how to make the response. The former concept was described as *selection*, the latter as *instruction*.

We now know that information to make specific immune responses does exist in the individual prior to the introduction of the antigen and that the antigen selects responses of the appropriate specificity. Determining how this occurs is one of the great stories of modern science. (See chapter 6 for a discussion of the experiments that established this and resolved the selection/instruction controversy.) The range of molecular configurations that can elicit immune responses is virtually unlimited; hence, the first law is *universality*.

The Law of Universality

The immune system is capable of making responses of great specificity. The range of substances against which antibodies can be made is virtually unlimited. As an illustration, it is at least theoretically possible to prepare a vaccine against any infectious agent. When the infectious agent for which the vaccine was designed enters the vaccinated individual, she or he responds much more vigorously than had the vaccine not been given. But that particular vaccine offers little or no protection against other infectious agents. Vaccination against smallpox provides robust protection against infection with the smallpox virus, but it does not offer protection against infection with measles virus; vaccination against measles virus does not protect us against the smallpox virus.

One way vaccines offer protection is by causing antibodies to form that react with and neutralize or lead to the destruction of the disease-causing microbe. The substance in the vaccine that elicits the immune response and for which the antibodies are specific is termed the *antigen*.[3] Vaccination also prepares the individual to make a secondary antibody response on infection with the microbe bearing the antigen or on rechallenge with the antigen or antigens that make up the vaccine. This secondary antibody response is much greater in amount and more rapid than the response would have been had the individual not been vaccinated. Responses to the first encounter with a vaccine or an infectious agent are designated *primary responses*.

The capacity of the immune system to make highly specific responses is so immense that under the proper circumstances, antibodies may be made that are specific to virtually any three-dimensional molecular structure. In principle, it is thus possible to make vaccines that would block the action of addictive drugs such as cocaine. Researchers have developed antibodies directed against molecules believed to be important in causing Alzheimer's disease. These antibodies are not yet successful in clinical trials, but they nonetheless show how broad the system of antibodies is in its capacity to be made against almost any molecular structure.

Antibodies are only one of the specificity elements of the immune system. As we have seen, the lymphocytes are equally important. These cells also display precise specificity for components of a vaccine, and the range of substance that may stimulate them to respond is comparable in its diversity to that of antibodies. This capacity for mounting immune responses of virtually any specificity is the law of universality.

The Law of Tolerance

Although the immune system can, in principle, make responses against a nearly boundless array of molecular configurations, there is a set of substances against which responses should not be made. These are the molecules that make up the body of the immunized individual, or the host. Responses against host tissue can be very destructive. When such responses do occur, the outcome is often an attack of immune cells against self-tissues that may result in the destruction of the tissue and thus the loss of its function. An example would be the development of type 1 diabetes due to immunologic destruction of insulin-producing cells in the pancreas.

Self-reactivity is prevented in most (but, unfortunately, not all) individuals by the operation of a series of mechanisms that together prevent the appearance or survival of potentially self-reactive lymphocytes or strikingly control such lymphocytes. These mechanisms that protect the body against potentially self-reactive lymphocytes are governed by the law of tolerance, which holds that the immune system does not attack the host.

The immune system must be able to distinguish between self-tissues and foreign substances. Self-tissues are generally ignored by the immune system, often as a result of mechanisms that lead to purging of the capacity to make specific self-reactions. If one attempts to produce antibodies by immunizing an experimental animal with its own proteins, generally little or no response occurs. But if a protein from a distinct species is used, then the animal makes a robust response, particularly if an ancillary stimulant, an adjuvant, is provided. When purging proves incomplete, other "backup" mechanisms are brought to bear that collectively suppress or regulate anti-self responses that might have occurred or are actually ongoing.

The Law of Appropriateness

The immune system has evolved a series of sensors that help it determine when it should mount a vigorous response against a foreign substance and when it should not. Mounting immune responses is energetically costly and if poorly regulated can be destructive to host tissues. The lymphocytes that respond may increase in frequency ten thousand times within a few days of a pathogen's detection. The products the immune cells make, while effective in controlling the infecting microbes, may lead to collateral tissue damage and inflammation. Although such energy expenditure and the damage that may occur is a small price to pay for protection against an infection with a virulent microorganism, they are unnecessary costs if the antigen-bearing substance poses no threat to the host.

To make certain that responses are only mounted when appropriate, a series of sensors of potentially pathogenic agents, mainly microorganisms, have developed. These sensors are called *pattern recognition receptors* (PRRs). The term was introduced by Charles Janeway of Yale University. He pointed out how important it was for the immune system to distinguish between antigenic substances that were innocuous and those that represented a threat. We now know of several different types of PRRs, but the first of these to be clearly recognized and to be studied in detail were toll-like receptors (TLRs) (see chapter 2). Janeway and his colleague, Ruslan Medzhitov, identified the first of these TLRs and some of the molecular pathways through which they mediate their function.

TLRs received their name as a result of their structural resemblance to toll, a molecule in the fruit fly, *Drosophila*. Jules Hoffmann and his colleagues in Strasbourg demonstrated that flies with mutations that prevented toll from functioning were unable to resist fungal infections, establishing that toll played an important role in fly immunity. Flies lack the lymphocyte/ antibody adaptive immune system that is so effective in humans and other vertebrates, but they do mount a robust innate immune response to potentially dangerous microbes. Toll is essential for the fly's innate immune response to certain classes of pathogens, most notably fungi.

Janeway proposed that the structures recognized by TLRs and other pattern recognition receptors be designated *pathogen-associated molecular patterns* (PAMPs). He argued that PAMPs would be molecules so central to the development and function of the microorganism that they could not easily be dispensed with. Janeway's vision was that the recognition of a PAMP by its complementary PRR would cause biochemical changes within the PRR-bearing cells. These changes would lead to expression of new genes and proteins that would aid lymphocytes that were specific for antigens of the microorganism to respond to that microorganism.

Janeway and Medzhitov showed that when TLRs on dendritic cells recognized the bacterial products for which the TLR was specific, the dendritic cells underwent a series of changes that resulted in their capacity to direct lymphocytes to mount a vigorous immune response. This is the same process that occurs when the immune system fights off Legionnaire's disease: dendritic cells move from the lung, where they take up legionella proteins, to the lymph node, where they present the antigenic fragments, together with MHC molecules, to T cells. By contrast, when PAMP recognition does not occur, the dendritic cells and other TLR-expressing "accessory" cells do not become activated and, in turn, the lymphocytes fail to make an effective immune response, even though there are among them cells that have the capacity to recognize the introduced foreign antigens.

The situation is certainly more complex than I have hinted at here. Different microorganisms live in different niches within the body (i.e., one infection differs strikingly from another in its location and in the cells and tissues involved). The effectiveness of immune system responses depends on the niches in which infectious agents establish themselves. The law of appropriateness determines whether a response should be mounted. Of equal importance is whether the response made is suitable to the threat posed by the microbe. In chapter 17, I discuss how the type of immune response may be tailored to the nature of the threat posed by the introduced pathogen.

The joint action of the three laws—universality, tolerance, and appropriateness—shapes the immune response. If the laws are "obeyed" and the threat posed by the infecting organism is not extreme, then in the vast majority of cases, the body handles infection well and the outcome is recovery. If the immune system is crippled for any reason, then vigorous and intensive treatment will be required and, even then, the outcome may be tragic.

4

Growing Up and Learning Immunology

My experiences in immunology have overlapped with, been illuminated by, and contributed to the amazing development of the field over the last five decades. Through sharing my own stories, I aim to give a more extended view of the laboratory experience itself and of the often complex process through which what we now regard as "truth"[1] is established.

I was born in Brooklyn, New York City. My father, Jack, had come to the United States as a teenager from a small town near Poltava in the Ukraine in 1913. My mother, Sylvia, was born in New York City. Her parents, William and Sadie Gleicher, had emigrated separately from Galicia in what was then the Polish portion of the Austro-Hungarian Empire and met and married in the United States.

My maternal grandmother Sadie's maiden name was Geschwind. Among my Geschwind cousins there were some quite well-known scientists. The most prominent was Norman Geschwind, who was the Putnam Professor of Neurology at Harvard Medical School and one of the founders of the field of behavioral neurology. His brother, Irving Geschwind, was an eminent hormone biochemist at the University of California, Davis. He had purified melanocyte stimulating hormone and established its relationship to adrenal cortical trophic hormone (ACTH), a subject that I would later work on briefly. Yet another cousin, Stanley Geschwind, was a distinguished physicist who was head of the quantum and solid-state physics department at Bell Labs for seventeen years.

My father owned an automobile repair business, and we lived in Brooklyn throughout my childhood. I attended New York City public schools, and like many other bright students in that era, I was pushed ahead so that

I graduated from high school at age sixteen. Looking back, I think I might have been better off moving along with others of my own age, albeit with a more enriched curriculum, but rapid promotion was the theory of the day. I attended Brooklyn College, where I majored in chemistry and was a premedical student. Brooklyn College offered an outstanding educational opportunity, and it was essentially free, representing New York City's investment in its next generation.

Medical school was at the State University of New York Downstate Medical Center, also in Brooklyn. There, in addition to the full medical school course, I had my first taste of research, working in the laboratory of one of my professors of anatomy, George Talbert. George was interested in protein hormones, like my cousin Irving Geschwind. He encouraged me to study the development of growth hormone production in the pituitaries of fetal and newborn rats. I learned a great deal from this initial foray into science, and it aided me when I later applied to a training position at the National Institutes of Health.

While in medical school I married Marilyn Heller, whom I had met while in college. Marilyn has been a mainstay of virtually all my efforts, and her judgment has been a sure guide for me. She remains the light of my life.

I did my internship and residency in internal medicine at the Massachusetts Memorial (Mass Memorial) Hospitals, then the main teaching hospital of the Boston University School of Medicine, where my cousin Norman Geschwind was a faculty member (prior to his appointment at Harvard). He and I met during my stay at Mass Memorial.

While I was doing my medical training at Mass Memorial, I joined the research lab headed by Alan Cohen in the Department of Medicine (figure 4.1). Alan was a leader in the study of amyloidosis, a disease in which proteins misfold and form fibrils whose deposition in various organs can lead to toxicity and loss of function in those organs. A component of amyloid is regarded as one of the inciting factors in Alzheimer's disease. At the time I was in Alan's lab, we did not know how the fibrils were formed or understand their chemical nature.

Alan had been studying the structure of amyloid fibrils using the high magnification that could be obtained with the electron microscope. I worked in his lab during a one-month elective and on nights and weekends while I was a resident. I took advantage of a new technology that allowed me to tag antibodies with ferritin, an iron-containing molecule that could

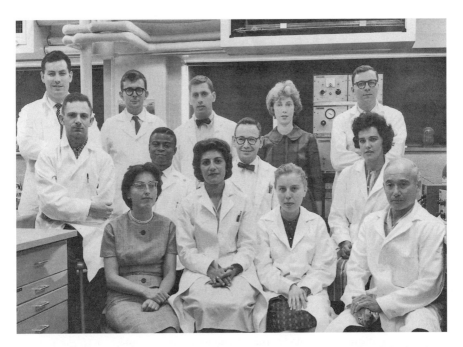

Figure 4.1. In Alan Cohen's laboratory in 1962. I am in the middle of the back row. Alan Cohen is third from the left in the second row. (Author's photo)

be visualized in the electron microscope. By using ferritin-labeled antibodies of different types, I could ask whether the antigen for which the antibody was specific was contained within the amyloid fibrils. That research led to my first two publications, one in *Nature* and the other in the *American Journal of Pathology*.[2]

In 1960, when I began my internship, young physicians in the United States were subject to being drafted into the armed forces. They could fulfill military obligation by being appointed to a position as a commissioned officer in the US Public Health Service and being assigned to NIH. Because such an appointment meant that the physician did not have to serve in the "real" military, and because NIH had an outstanding reputation for training young scientists, these appointments were highly sought after and quite difficult to get.

I applied to NIH, and in the fall of 1960, I was informed that I had been chosen for a position as a clinical associate in the Endocrinology Branch of the National Cancer Institute. The branch did both clinical and basic research. Its scientists studied the properties of various hormones and carried out clinical studies of patients with tumors of the endocrine system. I am sure that George Talbert's recommendation played an important role in my receiving one of these highly coveted positions.

It quickly became clear how important this NIH appointment was. In 1961, when I started my assistant residency in medicine at Mass Memorial, two out of the total of four assistant medical residents in my "class" were drafted. In that era, the practice was to draft the youngest men first. As I was just twenty-five, I surely would have been drafted had I not received the NIH appointment.

My two years at NIH, in Bethesda, Maryland, were a turning point. I was fortunate to have been there at a remarkable time. NIH had become the place for talented young physicians interested in science to train, and the success of that training is clear. In a recent article in *Science*, two eminent scientists, Joseph Goldstein and Michael Brown, pointed out that of the postdocs who trained at NIH between 1964 and 1972, nine would go on to win Nobel Prizes.[3] While not in that highly select group, I can testify to the excitement of the era and to the great achievement of so many of those who passed through NIH (and of many who stayed on).

While at NIH, I remained committed to clinical medicine as well as to research. The Endocrinology Branch offered an outstanding opportunity for one who wanted a mix of bench science and patient care. Roy Hertz, the branch chief, and M.-C. Li, a member of the branch who had moved on to the Memorial Sloan Kettering Cancer Center, had devised a curative therapy for choriocarcinoma, a malignancy of the placenta. "Chorio" was a relatively unusual tumor in the United States, although substantially more prevalent in other parts of the world. Virtually all the patients we saw were women in whom the malignancy had developed during pregnancy; they had metastatic disease, usually with enormous lesions in their lungs.

Hertz and Li had shown that administering the drug methotrexate in an aggressive regimen resulted in the cure of approximately 70 percent of their patients. For those of us who were privileged to care for these young women, it was an amazing clinical experience. The methotrexate cure of choriocarcinoma represents the first instance in which a metastatic malignancy could be routinely cured by drug therapy.

In parallel with my patient care responsibilities, I set up a research program aimed at studying the antigenic characteristics of key pituitary hormones. As part of this effort, I worked closely with Bill Odell, a principal investigator in the branch, and Jack Wilber, another clinical associate, to develop the first antibody-based assay for thyroid-stimulating hormone (TSH). Our assay allowed the accurate measurement of blood levels of this important pituitary hormone. The ability to measure the small amounts of TSH that were in the blood proved to be very valuable in the diagnosis of diseases of the thyroid, as well as pituitary abnormalities. The development of this assay was a major accomplishment, and the research paper describing it has been cited by other scientists more than five hundred times. Our research was based on earlier work by Rosalyn Yalow and Solomon Berson, who described the first radioimmunoassay, enabling them to measure blood levels for insulin.[4] Their work, done at the Bronx Veterans Administration Hospital in New York City, was eventually recognized with a Nobel Prize to Rosalyn Yalow, Berson having died in the interval.

I mentioned that my cousin Irving Geschwind had established that ACTH, the pituitary hormone that controls the production of steroid hormones by the adrenal gland, also could control the activity of melanocytes, the pigment cells of the skin. Bill Odell and I wanted to understand some of the key aspects of how ACTH mediated its activities both on pigment cells and on the adrenal. One of the key questions was whether the same portion of the ACTH molecule was required for the two functions.

At the time, one of the most powerful technologies to determine the size of a molecule that mediated a quantifiable function was to bombard that molecule with very high energy electrons and determine the amount of irradiation necessary to reduce the activity by a specific amount. The amounts of irradiation needed were large, as much as 600 million rads. The glass container in which the hormone was placed would become completely discolored from the intensity of the radiation. By way of comparison, the radiation dose in a typical chest X-ray is approximately 10 billion times less, about 0.06 rads.

We used a Van de Graff generator that NIH maintained in the basement of the hospital building for this and related purposes. The principle of the method was that if the emitted radiation were to cause an ionization within the volume of the molecule required for a given function, it would destroy the activity mediated by that molecular volume. We could calculate that volume from the dose of irradiation necessary to reduce activity by a particular amount (63.2%). We found, contrary to our expectation,

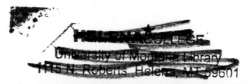

that the melanocyte stimulating activity of ACTH *increased* as we destroyed its adrenal stimulating activity, implying that some type of intramolecular inhibition was also part of the story. While we did not study this further, I felt a certain connection to this issue because it built on my cousin's earlier work.

My two years at NIH were truly eye-opening as they were my first real exposure to an outstanding research community. Our first son, Jonathan, was born while we were in Bethesda and, sadly, my father passed away just a few days before Jon's birth. While I found my NIH years exciting, I had already decided that what I really wanted to study was immunology, and I wanted to determine whether I could have a successful career as a research scientist.

I had been interested in immunology since my college days. Although immunology was definitely not included in the undergraduate curriculum in that era, at least not at Brooklyn College, I had come into the possession of a volume of essays by Michael Heidelberger. Heidelberger was one of the first scientists to place immunology on a quantitative basis, providing a key step in its transition from a set of observations to a coherent science. The book of his that I read described the remarkable specificity of antibodies and his efforts to understand the nature of the chemical bonds that formed between antigens and antibodies when they reacted with each other. I was completely captivated and became convinced that understanding the immune system represented a challenge that was worthy of a career.

Heidelberger had trained at the Rockefeller Institute (now the Rockefeller University) as a chemist and then as a postdoctoral fellow with the great biochemist Richard Willstätter in Munich. He spent the bulk of his active days as a professor at the Columbia University College of Physicians and Surgeons. Through one of those unusual twists that sometimes happen, when I came to New York University School of Medicine as a postdoctoral fellow in 1964, I worked in the lab that was immediately next to Heidelberger's. He had come to NYU in his second post-retirement position at the age of 75, and he continued to work there almost until the end of his life, at 104. I saw him almost daily for the four years I spent at NYU. He would often invite me to join him in a "gedanken" (thought) experiment, but we never did any "wet" experiments together.

As I had already decided I wanted to be an immunologist, while I was at NIH I applied to two of the most exciting scientists in the field, both based

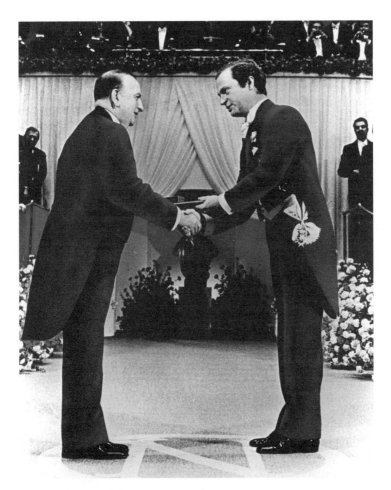

Figure 4.2. Baruj Benacerraf receiving the Nobel Prize from the King of Sweden in 1980. (Courtesy of the Dana-Farber Cancer Institute)

in New York City. They were Baruj Benacerraf, at NYU, and Henry Kunkel, at the Rockefeller University. Henry's lab was full, but Baruj was able to take me on.[5] This represented another of those fortunate events that determine the course of a life. Benacerraf would go on to win a Nobel Prize (figure 4.2), to be the chairman of the department of pathology at the Harvard Medical School, and to be the president of the Dana-Farber Cancer Institute at Harvard. However, these honors and responsibilities lay in the future. When I joined his lab, he was an up-and-coming scientist.

Baruj was born in Caracas, Venezuela, of Sephardic Jewish parents. His father was a successful businessman who had established an import company in Venezuela and set up a branch in France, moving with his family to Paris when Baruj was five. The Benacerrafs lived in Paris until 1939 when the coming of the war impelled Baruj's father to take the family back to Venezuela. Their stay in Caracas was brief because it was a priority that Baruj complete his education. The Benacerrafs came to New York City where Baruj first attended the École Française and then Columbia University. He met and wooed a young French woman, Annette Dreyfus, who had left Paris just before the fall of France. (Annette was distantly related to Captain Alfred Dreyfus, and her aunt had married Jacques Monod, the great French molecular biologist.)

After medical school, internship, and service in the US Army, Baruj began his career in immunology as a postdoctoral fellow with Elvin Kabat, a distinguished scientist, who had been Heidelberger's first PhD student, establishing yet another, albeit indirect, connection between myself and Heidelberger.

Completing his work at Columbia, Baruj returned to France, where he became a leader in the study of the biology of phagocytic cells (the cells that "eat" bacteria and particulate matter) in their normal setting in experimental animals. But after six years in Paris, Baruj found that he was still regarded as a foreigner in France, despite having grown up there, and he seized the opportunity to join the Department of Pathology at the NYU Medical School. At NYU, he established himself as a dominant figure, doing landmark studies in at least four different areas. It was here that he did the key work on the genetic control of immune responses that would lead to his Nobel Prize.

I arrived at the Benacerraf lab, room 527 of the NYU Medical Science Building, on July 1, 1964, eager and anxious to start my work, only to discover that Baruj was in Paris for the summer and that most of the other postdocs were on vacation. Fortunately, Ira Green, who was to become a lifelong friend, also had just arrived. We spent those summer days in 1964 thinking about the kinds of experiments that would help us to answer some of the central questions of immunology. I like to think that those discussions with Ira were critical to what was to come.

II THE FIRST LAW

Universality

5

Vaccines and Serum Therapy

Edward Jenner's experiment on Joseph Phipps showed how vaccination could protect against a potentially lethal infection. But it taught little beyond that because in 1796 there was no framework of knowledge of immunity, or of microbiology, within which to interpret the results. That would have to wait until the period of explosive scientific discovery during the last quarter of the nineteenth century, when Louis Pasteur and others put forth the germ theory of disease, recognized the immune response as an entity, and began to understand some of the principles of immunity.

Pasteur stated that chance favors the prepared mind—"*dans les champs de l'observation le hasard ne favorise que les esprits préparés.*"[1] He was well prepared for his own moment of serendipity. In 1880, he observed that cultures of the bacterium that causes chicken cholera[2] that had been inadvertently neglected over a holiday period failed to cause disease when inoculated into chickens. In the thriftiness that characterized scientific laboratories of that era, the chickens that had received the "defective" cultures of the chicken cholera bacteria were later used for other experiments. When these chickens were then challenged with virulent chicken cholera organisms, they proved to be resistant. Chickens that had not been previously inoculated with the weakened cultures, however, succumbed to the same dose of the virulent organism.

Pasteur immediately recognized the significance of this result. He had shown that introducing a weakened bacteria, one still capable of causing an infection but unable to cause disease or able to cause only mild disease, could induce a state of resistance in the individual that would protect against a later lethal challenge with bacteria of the same type. He understood that the *attenuated* chicken cholera bacterium had behaved much like vaccinia. Inoculating the weakened chicken cholera bacteria into chickens had caused an inapparent infection that resulted in the development of robust immunity just as vaccinia had done in inducing protection against smallpox infection.

Because of the seeming similarity in the mechanism of protection, Pasteur called his newly discovered process *vaccination* to honor Jenner's earlier contribution. The term originally developed to indicate inoculation with vaccinia to prevent smallpox has now been generalized to include all preventive immunizations. Today, vaccines are used to prevent a host of infectious diseases, and efforts to use vaccines in other settings, particularly as therapeutics for certain types of chronic infections, such as HIV, and for tumors, continue to be made.

Pasteur was not alone in exploring the capacity of bacteria and other microbes to cause disease and of vaccination to prevent them. A virtual scientific cataclysm occurred in the 1880s and 1890s, with amazing progress reported almost weekly. Anxious to prove the efficacy of the new science of vaccinology, Pasteur staged what is now a well-known public experiment.[3] He had developed an attenuated form of the bacteria that causes anthrax, a severe infectious disease of cattle, sheep, goats, and horses, which can also be lethal to humans. (In 2001, anthrax spores mailed to several US senators and news outlets resulted in five deaths.)

Pasteur vaccinated twenty-five sheep with his attenuated anthrax bacillus and left twenty-five untreated. Two weeks after a booster vaccine inoculation, on May 31, 1881, all fifty sheep were publically infected with lethal anthrax organisms at a farm in Pouilly-le-Fort, in Île-de-France, with local farmers, veterinarians, scientists, and the press in attendance. On June 2, the observers reassembled to assess the results, which precisely conformed to Pasteur's expectations. All but one of the unvaccinated sheep had died by the end of that day while all the recipients of the attenuated vaccine were healthy. The results were widely published, a public triumph for Pasteur personally as well as for the new science of vaccinology.

But even more public acclaim was to come. Pasteur attempted to develop an attenuated form of the virus that causes rabies by infecting rabbits with the "wild" rabies virus, isolating the virus from them, using it to infect another set of rabbits and continuing this "rabbit passage" through

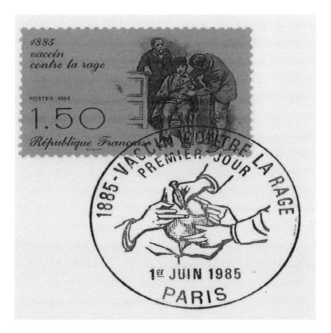

Figure 5.1. French postage stamp issued on the one hundredth anniversary of the inoculation of Joseph Meister with Pasteur's rabies vaccine.

many cycles in the expectation that the virus passed from rabbit to rabbit would lose its virulence for humans.

Pasteur showed that inoculation of the rabbit-passaged rabies virus protected dogs that were challenged with virulent rabies. Then on July 4, 1886, Joseph Meister, a nine-year-old boy, was severely bitten by a rabid dog. Without treatment (and there was no treatment at the time), he would almost surely have died. After much deliberation, Pasteur treated the boy with his preparation of attenuated rabies virus (figure 5.1). This virus preparation was in fact the dried spinal cord from rabbits in which the virus had been passaged.

Joseph Meister did not develop rabies. He lived until 1940 and, as an adult, worked as a caretaker at the Institut Pasteur in Paris, founded by Pasteur as a private nonprofit organization. It was the success of the rabies vaccine, more than anything else, that led to the virtual deification of Pasteur and the founding of more than twenty-five Pasteur Institutes throughout the world.

The successful development of vaccines to protect against infectious agents indicated that protective responses were not "flukes" that could only be developed against special types of organisms. Further, the protection provided by vaccines implicitly showed the specificity of immunity since it was necessary to use an attenuated form of a disease-causing organism in order to obtain protection against the virulent form of that organism.

Emil von Behring and his Japanese colleague Shibasaburo Kitasato at the Institute for Infectious Diseases in Berlin demonstrated the phenomenon of specificity more directly. Von Behring and Kitasato inoculated sterilized cultures of diphtheria or of tetanus organisms into horses, which caused these animals to produce substances that could neutralize the toxins made by the inoculated organisms. These substances, which could be obtained from the blood of the immunized horses, were called antitoxins.

Critically, antitoxins in the sera of diphtheria-immunized horses neutralized diphtheria toxin but not tetanus toxin whereas sera from the tetanus-immunized horses had the opposite effect. The sera containing these antitoxins were used to treat humans infected with diphtheria or tetanus organisms and were often successful in preventing the infected patient from succumbing to these toxins. For the development of *serum therapy*, von Behring, alone, received the first Nobel Prize in Physiology or Medicine, awarded in 1901. With the money from the prize, he established a pharmaceutical firm, Behringwerke, to produce the antitoxins. Behringwerke, located near the University of Marburg, where von Behring had been appointed professor of hygiene, eventually became one of the world's leading vaccine manufacturers. It was merged with the pharmaceutical giant Hoechst in 1952 and divided into components and sold in 1997.

6

How Is Specificity Achieved?

The demonstration that vaccination could prevent lethal diseases and that serum from vaccinated animals could prevent the damage caused by bacterial toxins was revolutionary. But scientists still needed an explanation for how immunization of animals caused the appearance of specific antitoxins and how introduction of an attenuated or an inactivated form of an organism elicited a specific protective response.

Ehrlich's Selection Theory

The eminent German scientist Paul Ehrlich developed drugs against syphilis and introduced the concept of chemotherapy (figure 6.1). He was a colleague of Emil von Behring in developing the antitoxins used to treat humans infected with the diphtheria bacterium. Indeed, it has been claimed that von Behring maneuvered to diminish the apparent importance of Ehrlich's contributions to the development of serum therapy to secure the Nobel Prize for himself alone.[1]

Ehrlich grappled with the problem of how the body distinguished one microorganism or one toxin from another. To explain this remarkable specificity, he proposed the idea that antibodies were cellular products that resembled the molecules on the surface of cells through which nutrients were imported. Ehrlich reasoned that each nutrient would be recognized by a distinct "nutrient receptor," and he argued that toxins were toxic because they could bind to nutrient receptors and prevent the receptors from being able to import nutrients into the cell. Each toxin would bind to a different nutrient receptor and thus be unique in its effects.

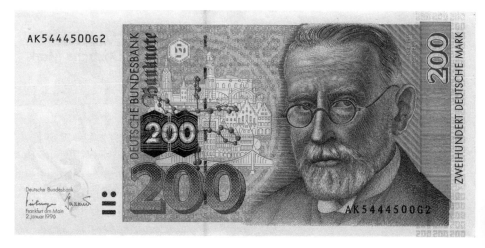

Figure 6.1. Paul Ehrlich on a German 200-mark note.

In Ehrlich's view, the immune response had evolved to counter the action of these toxins. He proposed that when a toxin bound to a nutrient receptor, and thereby prevented the import of a particular nutrient, the cell would respond by producing many more nutrient receptors of that particular type. These receptors occurred in the form of soluble molecules that could enter the blood. Thus, antibodies were in actuality soluble nutrient receptors. Being located in the blood, they would bind the toxin before it could reach the cell surface nutrient receptor and block its function. For this theory to be correct, it was necessary that the molecules that elicited antibody responses (antigens) were toxins. Because each toxin bound to a distinct nutrient receptor, the soluble nutrient receptors (antitoxins, antibodies) elicited by any given toxin would be different from those elicited by another toxin, accounting for the specificity of antibodies and for the immune response.

Ehrlich presented these ideas to the Royal Society of London in the prestigious Croonian Lecture in 1901. In that lecture, he proposed that cells "know" how to make antitoxins before they encounter the toxins that elicited their production. This proposition seemed reasonable because the antitoxin was actually the nutrient receptor in a somewhat different molecular form. Ehrlich argued that the toxin "selected" the appropriate antitoxin (antibody) response from among many potential responses that the cell already "knew" how to make. He also assumed that the cells that produced the antitoxin (recall that this was long before it was realized that these cells were lymphocytes) had the capacity to make antitoxins of many different specificities and that the toxin somehow determined which antitoxin the cell would make. He believed that the toxin (in modern terminology, the antigen) selected which antitoxin (that is, which antibody) would be produced. Critically, he indicated, too, that what was selected was the *antibody* itself.

While extremely prescient, Ehrlich's selection theory had a fatal flaw, which subsequent research would expose. The theory predicted that the universe of antigenic substances would be relatively limited, being confined to those molecules that could bind to nutrient receptors. It also held that antibodies were closely related to molecules that had a function distinct from being antibodies (i.e., they were soluble forms of nutrient receptors).

In addition, Ehrlich's theory could not readily explain why an initial contact with an antigen prepared an individual to make a more rapid and more vigorous response on subsequent encounter with the same antigen. This *memory response* partially explains the protection against infection that occurs as a result of vaccination and the similar (in practice, more robust) protection that develops in those who have experienced and recovered from a prior infection with the same microorganism. The failure of the Ehrlich selection theory to provide a reasonable explanation for memory would also lead to its falling out of favor.

Ehrlich was honored with the 1908 Nobel Prize, which he shared with Ilya Metchnikoff, for their "work on immunity." This prize honored the two distinct threads of immunology, innate immunity, which Metchnikoff studied, and adaptive immunity, Ehrlich's subject.

A Vast Antigenic Universe

To test Ehrlich's proposal, scientists needed a deeper understanding of the specificity of antibodies. They began to inject various substances whose chemical structure was well established into experimental animals in order to determine which elicited an antibody response and which did not. They also wished to learn whether the antibodies produced would discriminate between the substance used for immunization (the immunogen) and closely related chemical compounds.

The leader in this field was Karl Landsteiner (figure 6.2), a Vienna-born physician-scientist who discovered the ABO blood group substances and

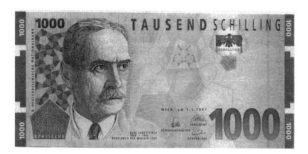

Figure 6.2. Karl Landsteiner on the Austrian thousand-schilling note.

thus was the father of blood transfusion. Landsteiner received the 1930 Nobel Prize in Physiology or Medicine for the discovery of blood group substances. With his colleague Alexander Wiener, he later co-discovered the Rh blood groups. Remarkably, Landsteiner also was the first to show that poliomyelitis was caused by an infectious agent. He successfully transmitted the disease to monkeys by injecting them with extracts of spinal cords from children who had died of polio.

After World War I, with Vienna reduced from the capital of the Habsburg empire to that of now-tiny Austria, opportunities for medical scientists there were limited. With a stopover in Holland, Landsteiner came to the United States to carry out his definitive studies of antibody specificity. He had been recruited to the Rockefeller Institute for Medical Research in New York City (now the Rockefeller University) by Simon Flexner, the first director of this world-famous institution.

The first observation Landsteiner and others made was that the injection of simple chemical compounds into experimental animals would generally not elicit the formation of antibodies. However, if the compound was chemically coupled to a protein molecule, injection of that complex would cause the formation of antibodies against the simple chemical (as well as against the protein). This discovery revealed that the capacity to elicit an immune response (to be an *immunogen*) was distinct from the capacity to react with antibodies. The modern term for a structure that can interact with an antibody is an *antigenic determinant*. An immunogen contains one or more antigenic determinants, but its immunogenicity stems from its ability to activate specific cells of the immune system.

By chemically attaching a very well defined small molecule to a protein and immunizing experimental animals with this conjugate, researchers

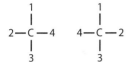

	Antigen contains	Antigen contains
Antiserum to:	L-tartaric acid	D-tartaric acid
L-tartaric acid	++	0
D-tartaric acid	0	++

Figure 6.3. Exquisite specificity of antibody responses. *Left*: optical isomers; two compounds are illustrated each with a central carbon atom (C). Carbon has the capacity to bind four substituents (1–4). The substituents can be arranged in two mirror image configurations. *Right*: antibodies discriminate optical isomers (L- and D-) of tartaric acid; degree of binding is indicated as ++ for strong or 0 for undetectable. (Adapted from K. Landsteiner and J. van der Scheer, *Journal of Experimental Medicine* 50 [1929]:407–17)

explored the precision of antigenic specificity. The protein to which the small molecule was attached would provide immunogenicity. If antibodies appeared that could react with (bind to) the small molecule by itself, then that molecule was regarded as containing an antigenic determinant. The term in general use for the small molecule is *hapten*, and that used for the protein to which the hapten was conjugated is *carrier*. The more "picturesque" German term *schlepper* is sometimes used for the carrier. Landsteiner obtained detailed information about the precision of antibody specificity by immunizing rabbits and guinea pigs with a variety of hapten-carrier conjugates. He showed that such specificity was exquisite. Antibodies could distinguish small molecules that differed from one another in very subtle ways.

Molecules, like parts of our bodies, can display the equivalent of handedness. That is, they can have the identical components but can be mirror images of one another rather than being superimposable. For example, if a single carbon atom can have four different atoms (or atom groups) associated with it, those groups can be arranged in such a manner that one form (isomer) will be a mirror image of the other (figure 6.3). These isomers often have the property that a solution of one will rotate a beam of polarized light in the clockwise direction while the other isomer will rotate light in a counterclockwise direction. Other than differences in how they rotate light, chemists often find it extremely difficult to distinguish such "optical" isomers from one another. But antibodies can distinguish these isomers virtually completely. As an example, tartaric acid displays optical isomerism, with the "L-isomer" rotating light in the clockwise direction and the D-isomer in the counterclockwise direction. Karl Landsteiner showed quite clearly that antibodies to L-tartaric acid do not bind to D-tartaric acid and vice versa.

Of equal importance, Landsteiner demonstrated that the universe of antigens was vast. Virtually any small chemical compound that he could attach to a suitable carrier protein would elicit a specific response when injected into an animal. Landsteiner synthesized compounds that, as far as could be judged, did not exist in nature. These compounds also contained antigenic determinants, as shown by the elicitation of specific antibodies when animals were immunized with these molecules conjugated to carrier proteins. The vastness of the antigenic universe was entirely at odds with Ehrlich's conception that antigens were largely limited to molecules that were toxins.

The realization about the size of the antigenic universe also challenged the idea that the information for making antibodies already existed in an individual before the immunogen that elicited those antibodies was inoculated (i.e., that the antigen selected a preexisting antibody). How would it be possible that the information to produce all these distinct antibody structures could already exist in the body at the time of immunization?

Landsteiner's work was carried out long before we understood the chemical basis of genetic information, although it was Oswald Avery, Landsteiner's colleague at the Rockefeller Institute, who established that DNA was the transmitter of such information. Because scientists lacked the detailed knowledge of how genes determined the structure of proteins, there was no means of testing whether the genetic information necessary to make all of the possible antibodies already existed in an individual before the injection of the immunogen. However, based on the enormous diversity of possible antibody responses, it seemed reasonable to conclude that antigen-mediated selection from a preexisting menu was very unlikely to be the basis of the immune response.

Instruction Theory

If antibodies (or the information to make them) did not preexist in the individual, then antigen could not select those antibodies with a good fit and cause them to be made in large amounts. How then did antigen elicit a specific antibody response? The obvious alternative was that the antigen provided the information needed for the production of specific antibodies.

Felix Haurowitz, a Czech biochemist, had been captivated by Landsteiner's study of antibody specificity. He took up Landsteiner's work and developed quantitative methods to measure the specificity of antibody with much greater precision. He was particularly interested in the antibody response to hemoglobin because he had been working on the structure of hemoglobin for much of his career. Haurowitz showed that the shape of hemoglobin crystals changed when they bound oxygen, a finding that inspired his subsequent work.

A cousin of Haurowitz's wife, Gina, was Max Perutz, an Austrian scientist, who visited the Haurowitzes on his way to England and was taken with Felix's demonstration of how oxygen affected the shape of hemoglobin crystals. Perutz took up the effort to solve the three-dimensional structure of hemoglobin in its forms both without oxygen and with oxygen. Perutz, who became one of the great stars of the Cambridge scientific community, was the founder of the modern science of protein crystallography, the determination of the structure of proteins using the diffraction of X-rays by the protein in a crystal form. He used this method to determine the detailed three-dimensional atomic structure of hemoglobin. He shared the 1962 Nobel Prize in Chemistry for this groundbreaking work.

Haurowitz meanwhile continued to investigate hemoglobin's properties for carrying information. He found that when hemoglobin bound oxygen, the shape of its crystal changed, which implied that small molecules bound to proteins could affect the structure of the protein. This realization led him to an entirely new theory of how antibodies were formed. Haurowitz proposed that the antigen "instructed" the antibody to attain its specificity. He argued that antibody molecules were synthesized in a largely floppy state, without a fixed three-dimensional structure. The antigenic determinant acted as a template around which the antibody folded, causing it to attain a structure in which the antibody was "complementary" to the antigenic determinant. The resulting folded molecule would retain its structure after it had dissociated from the "instructing" antigenic determinant (the template) and would thus be capable of binding new molecules bearing the same or a closely related antigenic determinant when they were introduced into the individual. Haurowitz's proposal became known as the *template theory*, an example of an instruction (as opposed to a selection) theory.

Haurowitz had carried out his research at the German University of Prague. In the summer of 1938, he was working at the Carlsberg Laboratory in Copenhagen when the Munich Agreement was signed, ceding the Czech region of the Sudetenland to Germany. Haurowitz immediately returned to Prague and, after a brief stint in the Czech army, found that he had been discharged from his professorship at the German University because he was Jewish. Fortunately, he received an offer from the University of Istanbul to be chairman of the biochemistry department there. He accepted and became part of a migration of Jewish academics to Turkey, where he and his colleagues survived the war and helped in the modernization of the Turkish universities.

The concept of instruction had some notable adherents. Linus Pauling, one of the greatest chemists of the twentieth century and a pioneer in the understanding of chemical bonds, championed the idea of instruction (figure 6.4). Pauling was by no means naïve regarding the structure of proteins. He discovered many of the key conformations that the amino acid chain adopted in folded proteins, such as the alpha helix. He received the 1954 Nobel Prize in Chemistry for his research into the nature of the chemical bond and the 1962 Nobel Peace Prize for his campaign against aboveground nuclear testing.

Pauling became interested in the problem of antibody specificity. Based on his deep knowledge of protein structure, he understood that the specificity of antibody molecules (i.e., their capacity to bind certain chemical compounds) was due to the details of their three-dimensional structure. He, too, could not see how the vast amount of information allowing the production of antibodies of essentially unlimited variability could exist in the body prior to immunization. As Haurowitz had done, Pauling became convinced that somehow the antigen dictated to the antibody its capacity to bind the antigenic determinant. He and his postdoctoral fellow Dan Campbell carried out some quite persuasive experiments at Cal Tech that appeared to support their ideas.

Pauling and Campbell prepared the fraction of the blood of an experimental animal known to be rich in antibodies and dissolved it in a solvent (urea) that would disrupt its conformation. This procedure caused the antibody molecules to attain a floppy structure similar, the scientists believed, to what they had before they encountered antigen. Pauling and Campbell then gradually removed the urea and included a test antigen in the solution. After several days with the urea completely removed, they also removed the test antigen and then asked whether this preparation could bind a new

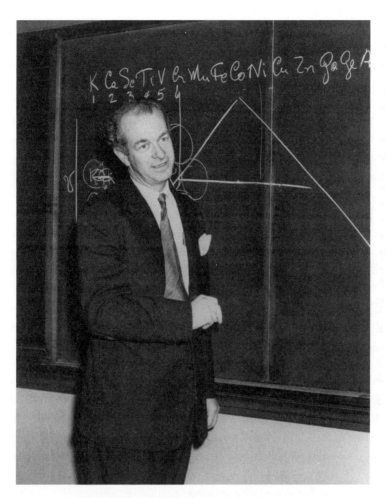

Figure 6.4. Linus Pauling lecturing in the 1940s. (Courtesy Ava Helen and Linus Pauling Papers, Oregon State University Libraries)

sample of the test antigen. To their satisfaction, it appeared to do so. Furthermore, although the antibody preparation could bind the antigen that had been present while the urea was being removed, it could not bind another antigen. It is now generally believed that there must be some other explanation for the result that Pauling and Campbell obtained because a vast body of data indicates that such antigen-directed folding does not occur in any meaningful way. Nonetheless, Pauling was sufficiently convinced by his work that he proposed that factories be set up during World

War II to use his new technology to produce antibodies that could be administered to soldiers who might be at risk of particular infections.

Instruction theories made certain clear predictions. Among them was that antigen should be present in antibody-producing cells to allow the instructive folding reaction to proceed. This presence could be tested if one could identify cells making a particular antibody and had a sufficiently sensitive assay for the antigen. But testing these ideas would have to await development of new technologies, and a more precise understanding of what exactly antibodies were. Progress on this front was made in the period immediately after the end of World War II.

Two of the most important names in deciphering the chemical nature of antibodies were Elvin Kabat and Michael Heidelberger. Heidelberger and Kabat had done work on quantitating antibody-antigen interactions, as had Haurowitz. Under Heidelberger's supervision at Columbia University, Kabat had prepared chemically purified antibodies. After earning his PhD in 1937, Kabat traveled to the University of Uppsala in Sweden to do a postdoctoral fellowship in the laboratory of Theodor Svedberg. There, Svedberg and his team were developing a series of instruments to analyze the structure of proteins. Working with Arne Tiselius, who had developed techniques for the preparative separation of proteins based on their electrical charge, Kabat showed that the purified antibodies he had made in Heidelberger's laboratory had a very specific mobility in an electrical field. Based on this mobility, they were designated *gamma globulins* (other proteins were said to have alpha or beta mobility), a term that continued in use for many years until replaced by the term *immunoglobulins*. This discovery paved the way for identifying antibody-producing cells.

I mentioned earlier that I was fortunate to have a connection with both Michael Heidelberger and Elvin Kabat through my being Baruj Benacerraf's postdoctoral fellow, he having been Kabat's postdoc, and Kabat having been Heidelberger's student. Also, I worked in the lab next to Heidelberger's at NYU for four years, seeing him almost every day.

After I moved from NYU to NIH, Akihiko Yano, a wonderful young Japanese scientist, joined my laboratory as a postdoctoral fellow. During Aki's stay in Bethesda, his wife gave birth to a son. Aki came to me to tell me it was a tradition for the "boss" to suggest a middle name for the baby. At first nonplussed, I soon concluded that Michael would be an appropriate name since Aki was my postdoc, I had been Benacerraf's postdoc, Benacerraf had been Kabat's postdoc, and Kabat had been Heidelberger's student. Accordingly, Dr. and Mrs. Yano named this little boy Takihiko Michael Yano.

Several weeks later, I attended a celebration of the hundredth anniversary of the NYU Department of Pathology. Michael Heidelberger was also in attendance. At the dinner, we were each asked to describe an anecdote that had some relevance to the department. I told the story of the naming of the Yanos's son. Michael was very pleased and shortly thereafter, the Yanos received a letter from Michael together with a check, asking them to start a bank account in Takihiko's name since Michael had done that with each of his grandchildren and wanted this young boy, who bore his name, to be similarly treated. Thereafter, letters were exchanged on Takihiko's birthday, and Aki translated Heidelberger's biographical articles into Japanese and arranged for their publication in a special issue of a well-known Japanese journal. At his hundredth birthday symposium, Michael's chief disappointment was that Aki was unable to be present.

The structure that Kabat and Tiselius had determined gave an important clue to understanding what cells made antibodies. It was known that there were human tumors that made gamma globulins. These tumors were *multiple myelomas*. Since multiple myelomas consist of malignant plasma cells, it seemed likely that normal plasma cells were the cells that physiologically produced antibodies, a conclusion that was being reached independently on morphological grounds by Astrid Fagreus working at the Karolinska Institutet in Stockholm. Knowing which cells made antibodies in general was important, but a method was needed to identify cells making an antibody of a particular specificity, that is, to identify the cells that were making antibodies that could bind a specific antigen.

Albert Coons at Harvard Medical School had been developing such a tool. He had realized that fluorescent compounds, such as fluorescein, which emits green light when exposed to blue light, could be used as markers if they could be attached to molecules that themselves would bind to cellular components. If a fluorescein-labeled antibody had bound to a constituent of the cells, then the cell would appear green under a fluorescence microscope when illuminated with blue light. While theoretically straightforward, putting all the pieces together was technically complicated. In

1940 and 1941, Coons collaborated with a graduate student, Ernst Berliner, from Louis Fieser's laboratory at Harvard Medical School. Fieser was one of the towering figures in organic chemistry, and Berliner was well suited to help Coons learn to make a derivative of fluorescein that contained a chemical grouping that allowed it to bind to proteins. Another colleague at Harvard, Allan Griffin, was in the process of assembling a microscope that could shine blue light on a sample and detect the green light emitted by compounds like fluorescein. This promising beginning, the account of which was published in 1941, had to be put aside during the war while Coons served for four years in the army in the South Pacific.

On returning to Harvard, Coons refined his work and made the technique practical. Eventually, he was able to conjugate fluorescein to an antigen so that he could detect cells making antibodies specific for that antigen since those cells, by having bound the fluorescein-antigen conjugate, would fluoresce when exposed to blue light in a fluorescence microscope.

As anticipated from the capacity of malignant plasma cells to make gamma globulin, Coons found that cells producing specific antibodies were largely plasma cells. However, only a small proportion of the plasma cells from an animal immunized with a conjugate of a fluoresceinated antigen were making an antibody capable of binding the fluoresceinated antigen. This finding assumed great importance later because it implied that antibody-producing cells were specialized to make a limited number of antibodies and thus the proportion of cells making a given antibody would be expected to be quite small.

Having found a method to detect cells producing specific antibodies, scientists needed a way to determine whether the antigen was also present in those cells. For this purpose, researchers used radioactive molecules. In one version of this experiment, carried out in John Humphrey's laboratory at the National Institute for Medical Research in Mill Hill, London, radioactive iodine (^{131}I) was incorporated into an integral component of the antigenic determinant such that it was essential for its binding to the antibody. Thus, if the radioactivity were not present, it would imply that the antigenic determinant was not there, at least to the limit of detection of the method. Very highly radioactive antigens were prepared so that the presence of very few molecules per cell could be detected. However, no evidence supporting the presence of antigen in antibody-producing cells was obtained. It was a strong argument against the instruction theory.

Primary Structure Determines Folded Structure

Instruction theories also failed as the understanding of how proteins assumed their final (folded) conformation progressed. The leader in establishing the principles underlying how proteins assumed their final shape was Christian Anfinsen. Anfinsen came from a family of Norwegian heritage and was raised in the Philadelphia area. He attended Swarthmore College and, while working for a master's degree in organic chemistry, received a scholarship to study at the Carlsberg Laboratory in Copenhagen. He arrived there in 1939, just a year after Haurowitz's tenure at the laboratory. Because of the war in Europe, Anfinsen returned to the United States in 1940, completed his PhD in biochemistry at Harvard Medical School, and was recruited to the National Heart Institute at NIH.

It was at NIH that he did his pathbreaking experiment establishing that the three-dimensional structure of proteins was determined by the linear order of their constituent amino acids. Anfinsen analyzed the activity of an enzyme from staphylococcal bacteria that could cleave ribonucleic acid (RNA). The folded structure of this enzyme, staphylococcal ribonuclease, was, in part, determined by cross-linkages within the protein between cysteines, sulfur-containing amino acids. These *disulfide bonds* represented linkages of the sulfur atom of one cysteine to the sulfur atom of another. Staphylococcal ribonuclease contained eight cysteines and, in principle, could adopt twenty-eight distinct patterns of cross-linkage if the folding of the protein was a random process and thus if the cysteines that bound to one another were not predetermined.

Anfinsen first broke the disulfide bonds between cysteines using chemical methods and then used urea to unfold the molecule, just as Campbell and Pauling had done in their experiments. The unfolded molecule lost all of its capacity to cleave ribonuclease. Anfinsen then allowed the molecule to refold spontaneously and to reform its disulfide bonds by removing the urea and subjecting the protein to mild oxidizing conditions. As only the enzyme with the original pattern of disulfide bonds would regain the capacity to cleave RNA, he reasoned that he could estimate the degree of refolding to the original conformation of the protein by determining the amount of enzymatic activity of the reoxidized protein.

Anfinsen and his postdoctoral fellow, Ed Haber, observed that the original structure was reformed preferentially; the enzyme activity was more than fifteen times that predicted if refolding had been random. This result led Anfinsen to formulate the concept that the three-dimensional structure of proteins was determined by the linear order of the amino acids (their primary structure). The idea is often referred to as Anfinsen's dogma. For this work, Anfinsen received the 1972 Nobel Prize in Chemistry.

If primary structure determined folded structure, then it should not be possible for the presence of different antigenic determinants around which the protein could fold to confer distinct specificities on an identical set of antibody molecules.

Anfinsen was a towering figure at NIH. I remember him quite well (figure 6.5). Although one of the most distinguished scientists in the world, he was very approachable and cared deeply about students and postdocs. I can recall attending evening events in which he spoke with groups of medical students that the Howard Hughes Medical Institute had brought to

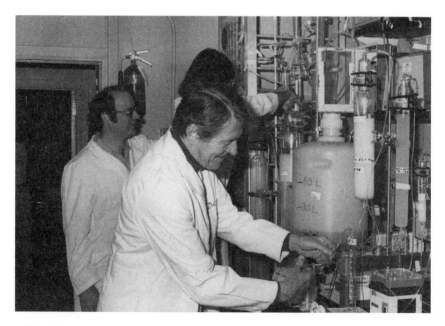

Figure 6.5. Christian Anfinsen working in his laboratory at NIH. (From the Christian B. Anfinsen Papers, National Library of Medicine)

NIH for a year. Anfinsen was the ultimate civilized individual, deeply knowledgeable, open to discussion, and truly interested in younger people.

Having suffered the blow of the lack of antigen in antibody-producing cells and going against Anfinsen's dogma, the template theory did not survive. In addition to these experimental challenges to instruction, the template theory was not very useful in explaining the biology of the immune response. It offered no simple explanation for immunologic memory, since newly synthesized antibody molecules would have to be folded by antigen during secondary responses just as they had during primary responses.

7

Immunology's "Eureka"

Clonal Selection

The failures of instruction theory and Ehrlich's selection theory left immunology without a viable framework within which to understand immunological specificity and immunological memory. Furthermore, there was a growing recognition that non-antibody-based specific immune responses, *cellular immune responses*, were of great importance, yet theory had largely ignored them. Clearly, an entirely new approach was needed.

Selection Returns

The first to reconsider selection as a basis for immune responses was Niels Jerne, in 1955, when he was working at the Danish National Serum Institute in Copenhagen. Jerne was remarkably prescient throughout his scientific career. He would identify a critical problem early, make a provocative proposal to illustrate the centrality of the idea, and attract others to attack the problem in detail. In the reintroduction of selection, the analysis of the role of the thymus in development of T-cell specificity, and the concept that antibodies are involved in a network of mutual interactions, Jerne's initial ideas were rather off the mark. Nevertheless, his proposals galvanized the field and eventually led to a deeper understanding of immunologic specificity, immune tolerance, and immune regulation. Jerne received the 1984 Nobel Prize for Physiology or Medicine. The citation emphasized his contributions to the development of modern selection theories; however, the modern selection theories that form the theoretical underpinning of contemporary immunology would be introduced not by Jerne but by David Talmage and Macfarlane Burnet.

In a 1955 paper, Jerne proposed that antibodies specific for most compounds preexisted in the body prior to immunization (he termed them *natural antibodies*) and circulated in the blood.[1] Jerne argued that when an antigen was introduced, it would rapidly bind to an already existing natural antibody and the resultant antigen-antibody complex would be transported to cells potentially capable of producing antibodies. The antigen-antibody complex would elicit the production of precisely those antibodies that were contained within the complex. This required that the cell had a mechanism through which it could recognize which antibody was in the complex and would cause the production of more of the same antibody. By inference, his theory, designated *natural selection*, also implied that each cell could make many different antibodies and which antibody it made was determined by the antibody in the antigen-antibody complex.

Some have regarded natural selection as simply a reworking of Ehrlich's selection theory, and several of its elements are indeed similar. However, Jerne made some important changes to Ehrlich's ideas. He abandoned the notion that antibodies were soluble nutrient receptors, and he accepted that the antibody universe was very large. However, the major flaw in Jerne's natural selection theory is that it retained Ehrlich's view that antigen (or antibody) selected the antibody and that the antibody (not the cell producing it) "expanded" on priming.

Talmage, Burnet, and Cell Selection

In 1957, David Talmage, then a young faculty member in the Department of Medicine at the University of Chicago School of Medicine, and Macfarlane Burnet, the director of the Walter and Eliza Hall Institute in Melbourne, independently proposed an explanation for the immune response that was radically different from all prior ideas and based on a deep appreciation of the biological principles of immunity, most importantly on the need to account for immunological memory and for immunological tolerance.

Talmage and Burnet postulated that individual lymphocytes could make responses of only a single specificity. They argued that the vast potential of the immune system was accounted for by the presence of an extremely large number of lymphocytes, each with a specificity that was unique, or at least shared by a relatively small number of other cells. Recall that only a small proportion of antibody-producing cells make antibody to any given antigen.

In the Talmage-Burnet view, the specificity of individual lymphocytes was based on the expression on their surface of receptors that could bind only a limited number of structurally related antigenic determinants. Encounter with antigen led to an appropriate response because the antigen selected those rare cells with receptors specific for it. In the case of B cells, those cells with specific receptors could then produce antibodies of the same limited specificity. Although superficially, these ideas seem similar to those of Ehrlich's, there are key differences. Those differences resulted in Talmage and Burnet's concept providing us with a theoretical basis for understanding of the biology of immunity.

Ehrlich believed that each cell had many different receptors and could make many different antibodies. Of these many potential antibodies, antigen selected what a cell actually produced. Jerne's natural selection theory shared this central idea. Both Ehrlich and Jerne shared the assumption that antigen determined which of the many antibodies an individual cell *could* make, it actually *would* make. Thus, what was selected by the antigen was the antibody.

Talmage and Burnet, by contrast, argued that each cell could make but a single antibody and that each cell had receptors of only one specificity, equivalent to that of the antibody it could make. The process of binding antigen to the receptor of a lymphocyte resulted in the transmission of a biochemical signal into the cell. The signal caused that cell both to divide and to undergo a set of differentiation events that would prepare it to mediate functions that protected the body against the invading microorganisms expressing that antigen. Responding B cells would develop into antibody-producing cells; T cells could acquire the capacity to kill infected cells or to make potent effector molecules, such as cytokines, that could help to control the pathogen. An alternative outcome of antigen encounter could be the elimination or inactivation of the receptor-bearing cell.

Thus, the critical distinction Talmage and Burnet introduced was that antigen selected a cell, not, as in Ehrlich and Jerne's concept, a nonliving entity, an antibody. The cell's capacity to divide and thus increase in number, to change and acquire new functions, or even to be eliminated could explain the biological properties of the immune response.

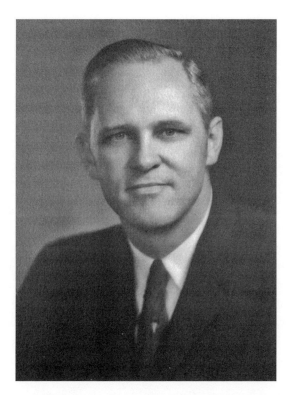

Figure 7.1. David Talmage. (Courtesy of Marilyn Talmage-Bowers)

David Talmage was born in Korea in 1919 (figure 7.1). His parents were Presbyterian missionaries who were "teachers and preachers" in Kwangju in what is now South Korea. Talmage's early schooling was in Kwangju, but later he attended the Pyeng Yang Foreign School, an American Presbyterian Mission School in the city that is today the capital of North Korea. Talmage came to the United States to attend Davidson College in North Carolina. He then enrolled in the Washington University School of Medicine in 1941.

Just a few months later the country was at war, and Talmage was inducted into the US Army and completed medical school in three years as a private. After a shortened internship, he was assigned to duty in the Philippines but learned that there was a cholera epidemic in Korea and persuaded his commanding officer to transfer him to Korea where, based on his knowledge of Korean, he felt he could do the most good.

After completing his military service, Talmage served a second internship at Barnes Hospital in St. Louis and fell under the tutelage of Frank Dixon, a wunderkind of the study of the mechanisms through which the immune system causes tissue damage. Though Talmage followed Dixon to Pittsburgh, he then struck out on his own, moving to the Department of Medicine at the University of Chicago. There, he became interested in two quite distinct problems: the effect of X-rays on the immune system and the enormous diversity of antibody molecules. It was the integration of these disparate interests that led him to what he called *cellular selection*.

Working with colleagues, Talmage had shown that exposing a mouse to X-rays before immunization would prevent an antibody response whereas delaying the exposure for several days after immunization would have a much more limited effect. It was known that dividing cells were particularly sensitive to X-rays, so this result suggested that cell division was required for an organism to make an antibody response. Delaying irradiation did not interrupt antibody production presumably because the divisions of the cell that was to produce antibody had largely been completed by the time of delayed exposure to X-rays. Thus, Talmage and his colleagues concluded that cell division was an essential feature of antibody responses.

Talmage also rejected all theories that required that antibody molecules be altered by interaction with antigen, and he found it implausible that a cell could preferentially produce a single antibody out of many based on the introduction of a few copies of that antibody, as Jerne's natural selection theory implied. His work on antibody diversity had shown the vastness of the universe of antibodies, and it led him to the conclusion that the antigen selected cells with antibodies on their surface that could bind the antigen. Moreover, he realized, the immune response was specific because each cell expressed cell surface antibodies of one type only. After the cell had produced many copies of itself through cell division, those cells would secrete antibodies essentially identical to their surface antibodies except that they were soluble and could thus enter the blood and the tissue fluids rather than being confined to the cell surface.

Talmage not only had a distinguished career as a medical researcher but also, remarkably, after retirement turned his attention to fundamental problems of physics. One of his last publications was "A Biologist's

Struggle with the Physics Problem: General Relativity Theory and Quantum Mechanics Are Incompatible." David Talmage died on March 6, 2014, at the age of ninety-four.

A final note about Talmage. After publishing his cellular selection theory, he did not remain long at the University of Chicago but was recruited to the University of Colorado School of Medicine in Denver. A few years ago, I was asked to give the opening lecture at the "retreat" of the immunology graduate students at the University of Chicago. I chose for my topic the development of ideas in immunology. To my surprise and chagrin, none of the students and, as far as I could tell, few of the immunology faculty were aware that Talmage's landmark contribution to immunology was made while he was a University of Chicago faculty member. No plaque marking this accomplishment existed. Of course, his contribution does not require that type of "laudation," but I would think his accomplishment would be an inspiration to young University of Chicago students and trainees in our field.

Macfarlane Burnet suffers no such lack of remembrance among Australians, who still refer to him as "Sir Mac." More than fifty years after proposing his theory of clonal selection and long after his death, Burnet remains a towering figure in the Australian scientific community.

Talmage's description of cellular selection was published in the *Annual Review of Medicine* in early 1957. Burnet already had been thinking along similar lines, and his clonal selection theory (same idea, different name) was published in October 1957 in the *Australian Journal of Science*. In contrast to Talmage, who was young and not widely known, Burnet was a scientific giant even before clonal selection.

Frank Macfarlane Burnet (figure 7.2) was born in 1899 in Taralgon, Victoria. He received his medical degree from the University of Melbourne and began his research career at the Hall Institute in 1923, studying typhoid fever. From 1925 to 1928, he studied in London, still working on bacteria, and received a PhD from the University of London. Returning to Australia, he was appointed deputy director of the Hall Institute. A second stint in London, at the National Institute for Medical Research from 1933 to 1934, turned his research interests to the study of viruses. Back again at the Hall Institute, he worked on several subjects, including viruses transmitted by parrots and cockatoos and the bacterial infection known as Q fever, for

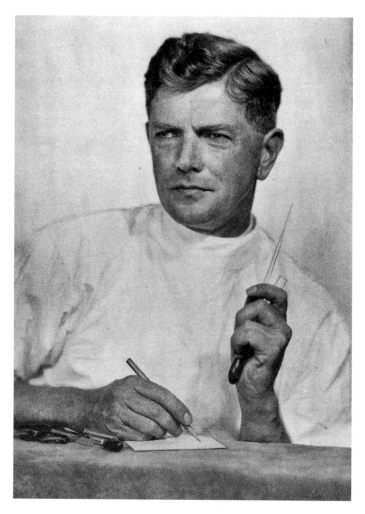

Figure 7.2. Frank Macfarlane Burnet ("Sir Mac") at work. (Courtesy of the Walter and Eliza Hall Institute for Medical Research)

which he discovered the causative agent, named in his honor as *Coxiella burnetii*. Burnet was appointed director of the Hall Institute in 1944, a post he held until his retirement.

Burnet again changed his interests, this time to immunology, and his writings on the production of antibodies were influential, as were his ideas about immunological tolerance and his views on the ability of the immune system to distinguish self from nonself tissues. Indeed, it was for his proposals about tolerance (which I discuss in chapter 13) that he was awarded the Nobel Prize in 1984.

Burnet's paper in the *Australian Journal of Science* in late 1957 represented his co-proposal of clonal selection. But what truly established the close identification between Burnet and clonal selection (much more than with Talmage) was his publication in 1959 of *The Clonal Selection Theory of Acquired Immunity*.[2] In this book, Burnet masterfully explained the concept and its implications in detail and showed how the theory could account for a vast amount of data concerning the biology of immune responses that no prior theory had done with any degree of success. I recall reading Burnet's book when I entered Baruj Benacerraf's laboratory in 1964 and being immensely impressed by the depth of Burnet's vision of how clonal selection explained virtually every aspect of immunology. It can be argued that clonal selection is to immunology as Darwinian evolution is to biology in general.

Burnet's term, *clonal selection*, lives on, although I believe Talmage's *cellular selection* is a better name. Clonal selection is somewhat misleading because it implies that the key event is the selection of a clone (a population of identical cells). What antigen actually selects on being introduced into the body are individual naïve cells. The cells may then form clones as a result of explosive antigen-driven cell division. However, clonal selection remains the term used. As a theory, clonal selection has proven remarkably robust. It provides the framework with which to understand virtually all aspects of modern immunology.

The Clonal Selection Theory

The clonal selection theory holds that lymphocytes have cell surface receptors that allow them to recognize and respond to antigen and that each lymphocyte has a population of receptors that all have the same binding specificity (figure 7.3). The large size of the antigenic universe implies that the number of lymphocytes with receptors of distinct specificity must be very large and the frequency of lymphocytes with any particular specificity correspondingly small. Current estimates of the frequency of lymphocytes specific for common antigens in a previously unimmmunized individual range from one per hundred thousand cells to one per million cells. However, the proliferative potential of lymphocytes when they have encountered an antigen for which their receptors are complementary, and

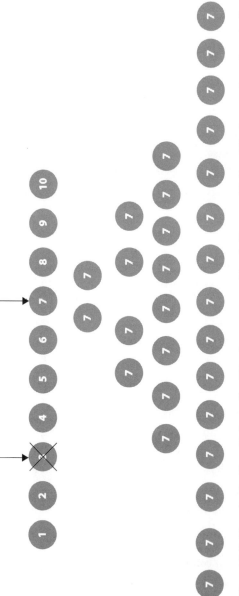

Figure 7.3. Clonal selection. Naïve cells differ from one another in the specificity of their receptors, here indicated by different numbers. When an antigen interacts with a naïve cell whose receptor can bind the antigen (cells 3 and 7), the cell may be stimulated to divide and form a large clone (cell 7). Under other circumstances, the interaction may lead to the elimination of the cell, a phenomenon known as deletional tolerance (cell 3).

when that encounter has occurred under appropriate conditions, is enormous. Viral infection may cause precursors of killer T cells specific for antigens of that virus to expand ten-thousand-fold within a week of infection. Thus, in a relatively short time after antigen encounter, the rare cells specific for a particular viral antigenic determinant may expand in number sufficiently so that they constitute as many as 10 percent of the cells of their type or even more. If all goes well, they and their products can completely eliminate the microbial pathogen.

Burnet emphasized that the optimal form of the clonal selection theory required that the receptors be distributed one specificity to a lymphocyte. Also, for B cells, the specificity of the receptor and that of the antibody produced by the clonal descendants of the initially responding cell should be the same. These conditions would ensure that only antibodies capable of reacting with the inciting antigen be produced and that the elimination of self-reactive cells would not also lead to the elimination of cells capable of reacting against foreign substances. Although we now know it to be somewhat of an oversimplification, this concept has great power in helping us understand the biology of the immune system and make predictions about how that system will behave under new circumstances.

In its simplest form, clonal selection envisages the lymphocyte population as essentially equivalent to a population of unicellular organisms living within us. The lymphocytes undergo a process of natural selection, à la Darwin: those with a reproductive advantage (i.e., the capacity to bind to and be stimulated to proliferate by antigen) achieve dominance. This process, of course, takes place within the lifetime of an individual and is not transmitted to his or her offspring (it occurs in lymphocytes, not in sperm or egg cells), so that for the immunized individual it may be regarded as *somatic evolution*, although for the lymphocytes themselves it represents the more conventional Darwinian evolution.

The analogy between individual lymphocytes and unicellular organisms should not be taken too far as there are very substantial homeostatic controls that determine the overall size and makeup of the lymphocyte population. However, the "lymphocyte as unicellular organism" notion illustrates how the immune system can cope with an unpredictable and ever-changing microbial world.

For B cells, there is a further twist to the process of selection and expansion. In the course of responding to a particular antigen, the B lymphocytes with receptors specific for that antigen not only proliferate vigorously but also activate a mechanism that results in an extremely high rate of mutation in the genes that specify the antibody. This process, *somatic hypermutation* (SHM), results on a new genetic pool in which selection can continue to operate, thus leading to an even greater degree of evolution of the B lymphocyte population in response to ongoing antigenic stimulation. The B cells that are selected are ones whose receptors bind to the antigen most tightly, and thus late in an immune response, the specific B cells and the antibody they produce, bind the antigen much more tightly than they do early in the response. For that reason, even very small amounts of antibody present in an individual that was immunized in the past can be very effective in neutralizing a microbe.

The Impact of Clonal Selection

The proposal of the clonal selection theory led to an enormous burst of research that resulted in the development of a new subfield of immunology, *cellular immunology*. One of the immediate goals of cellular immunology was to test the concept that an individual cell had a single specificity. At that time, the nature of receptors for antigen had not yet been determined. Even the distinction between B and T lymphocytes had not been established. The obvious question was to ask whether in an individual immunized with more than one antigen did antibody-producing cells produce one or more than one type of antibody. According to the theory, lymphocytes would have receptors of only one specificity so that the antibody-producing descendants of a precursor B cell should only produce antibodies specific for the antigen that stimulated the precursor cell, and all the antibodies made by an individual member of the resultant clone should be the same. Of course, the operation of SHM would lead to different cells derived from the same precursor (different members of the clone) making somewhat different antibodies since a mutation in one cell would alter the antibody it produced. Nevertheless, that cell should still produce a homogeneous set of antibodies, although they would differ from the antibodies made by the clonal progenitor due to the mutations that had occurred.

The task of determining whether all the antibody proteins an individual antibody-producing cell made were the same was not within experimental reach at the time clonal selection theory was introduced. However, there were experiments that provided powerful supporting evidence. The analysis of the proteins made by multiple myeloma cells (or by experimental tumors of antibody-producing cells in the mouse, called plasmacytomas) revealed that these proteins had the structure of antibodies and that the myeloma proteins (antibodies) produced by individual tumors were usually homogeneous.

An alternative strategy was to immunize an experimental animal with two antigens and ask whether individual cells made antibodies specific for each antigen or for only one of the two antigens. The most influential experiment aimed at testing this was performed by Gus Nossal, a protégé of Burnet and his successor as director of the Hall Institute, and Joshua Lederberg, a wunderkind who had received a Nobel Prize at the age of thirty-three for his epic studies in bacterial genetics.

Lederberg had become interested in the antibody problem, recognizing, like Talmage and Burnet, that it was an issue of cellular selection, not antibody selection. He took a sabbatical at the Hall Institute from his position at the University of Wisconsin. There, he and Nossal immunized rats with two different strains of the salmonella bacteria. Antibodies directed at the flagella (whiplike appendages the bacteria use to move) of the different strains of salmonella can be detected because they immobilize the bacteria. Nossal and Lederberg placed individual antibody-producing cells within microdroplets and introduced both strains of bacteria into each droplet. By 1958, they had observed that only one strain of the bacteria was immobilized in any individual droplet. This indicated that in an animal immunized with two antigens, individual cells made antibody to only one of the two antigens; some made antibody to one, some to the other, and many to neither.

Some years later, while I was in the Benacerraf laboratory, Ira Green and Baruj, working with Pierre Vassalli, carried out an experiment in which they directly visualized the antibodies produced by individual cells from animals immunized with several antigens. They showed that virtually none of the antibody-producing cells made antibodies directed at more than one of the antigenic determinants that had been used for immunization.

Such tests, however, did not completely prove that individual cells made antibodies of only a single specificity, only that individual cells did not make a large number of different antibodies. Because the frequency of cells making antibody for any given antigen is generally quite low, the chance that a cell will have two such specificities is small even if the cells could produce more than one antibody. For example, even if an individual cell can make more than one antibody, if an animal is immunized with antigen A and antigen B and the frequency of cells producing anti-A and anti-B are each one per hundred (actually quite a high frequency), then only one-hundredth of the anti-A producing cells would also be producing anti-B and vice versa.[3]

Taking this discussion a step further, one can imagine that a clonal selection process might work quite well as long as an individual cell could only produce a small proportion of the potential antibodies that the entire system could make or express a small proportion of potential T-cell receptors, particularly if the patterns of co-expression were random. This would still yield responses that had a high degree of specificity and would account for immunologic memory, and the loss of "foreign-reactive potential" as a result of eliminating self-reactive cells would be modest.

Modern technology allowing the analysis of proteins and genes expressed in individual cells has provided powerful confirmation that the great majority of B lymphocytes express only a single receptor and that each of their clonal descendants make antibody of one structure and one specificity. By contrast, T cells not uncommonly express two TCRs of different specificities. However, that the system has come very close to the simple version of clonal selection strongly suggests there is a substantial survival advantage in doing so. Several advantages have been suggested, but the most compelling is the limitation in autoreactivity achieved by preventing the expansion and differentiation of cells with receptors specific for a foreign antigen that also have receptors specific for a self-antigen. If a cell specific for both a self and a foreign antigen somehow escaped elimination (there are potent mechanisms to eliminate self-reactive cells, which I discuss in detail later), the activation of that cell by the foreign antigen for which it is specific could result in an attack on tissues expressing the self-antigen for which the cell is also specific. It can be argued that to make this unlikely, the system evolved close to the one-specificity-to-one-cell limit.

Clonal selection is attractive because it explains not only immunologic memory (i.e., the heightened response seen in antigen-experienced individuals based on the prior expansion and differentiation of antigen-specific cells during a primary response) but also the lack of response to the antigens of self-tissues. As I discuss in the next chapter, the process through which developing lymphocytes acquire the particular cell surface receptors they will express as mature cells has a large random component. Thus, some (perhaps many) developing lymphocytes can be expected to express receptors that are specific for antigens expressed by the individual in whom they develop. Burnet and Lederberg independently recognized that if mechanisms existed to test the specificity of lymphocytes by exposing them to self-antigens at a critical stage of their development, these lymphocytes could be eliminated at that time and thus would pose no threat to the individual. We now know that such a process does take place. For T lymphocytes, cellular elimination occurs during development within the thymus, so that the population of T lymphocytes emerging from the thymus and entering the peripheral lymphoid organs has been purged of many cells that would have been self-reactive had they not been eliminated.

This elimination process is only one of several mechanisms that have developed to prevent or control self-reactivity (or autoreactivity) and thus to prevent autoimmune disorders. However, these control mechanisms, while very efficient, are not perfect, and autoimmune responses and autoimmune diseases such as type 1 diabetes do occur.

Thus, the clonal selection theory provides immunologists with an elegant and comprehensive structure that can provide explanations for virtually all of the biologic properties of immunity and, most importantly, could guide researchers to undertake the experiments that would provide detailed cellular and molecular mechanisms for the normal function of the immune system and for its disordered function in autoimmunity and immunodeficiency. Indeed, the modern introduction of potent drugs to treat immunologic diseases or to restore immunity to tumors could hardly be imagined outside of the context of this theory.

8

How Does Each Lymphocyte Develop

a Distinct Receptor?

The majority of the immunology community quickly embraced clonal selection. The theory provided a powerful explanation of the biology of immune responses, and experiments demonstrated that individual cells from animals immunized with several antigens rarely if ever made antibodies specific for more than one antigen.

But within the clonal selection proposal were big unanswered questions. Where did the information encoding all these specificities come from, and what process segregated the specificities one to a cell? Talmage and Burnet did not consider these issues explicitly, but once clonal selection theory was generally accepted, resolving these points became the dominant scientific challenge facing immunologists.

Scientists had rejected Ehrlich's selection theory in part because it could not account for the vast size of the universe of antigens and the similarly vast set of complementary antibodies and T-cell receptors needed to recognize these antigens. One view put forward was that the information required to produce all the antibodies, or B-cell receptors (BCRs), and all the T-cell receptors (TCRs) was transmitted genetically. That is, each BCR and TCR was encoded in a conventional gene that existed in the genome and was handed down from parents to children in a normal manner. Since the number of distinct TCRs and BCRs is believed to be in the millions, a comparably large number of TCR and BCR genes would have to exist. According to this view, the determination that each T cell and each B cell expressed only a single TCR or BCR was a matter of differentiation. As each cell developed, it would choose to activate only one of the vast number of different BCR or TCR genes present in its genome (and in the genome of every other cell in the body), possibly on an entirely random basis.

This *germline* theory had the virtue of straightforwardness, but, in its simplest form, it required that an enormous proportion of the genome be given over to coding for BCR[1] and TCR genes. Indeed, we now know that humans have approximately 25,000 genes. That means that the entire genome is insufficient to encode all the antibody and TCR genes required for the expressed repertoire.[2]

The alternative theory held, in its most extreme form, that there was only a single gene encoding BCRs, another encoding TCRs, and that there was a very active process of mutation in individual clonal precursors that led to the diversification of these genes so that each precursor ended up with a distinctive BCR/antibody gene or a distinctive TCR gene. This theory was dubbed the *somatic mutation* theory.

Trying to resolve which theory, or combination of theories, actually explained the observed large universe of receptors and their segregation one (or occasionally two) to a cell dominated immunological science for a decade. By the time this controversy was at its height, the process of determining the sequence of amino acids in proteins had been improved, and scientists had determined the precise order of amino acids in the polypeptide chains of many different antibodies. Efforts to understand the process of receptor diversification and segregation based on the analyses of these sequences produced much heat but, with a few exceptions, little light.

Solving the problem of the genetic basis for diversification awaited the development of the modern tools of molecular biology that allowed genes to be identified and characterized. Techniques had been developed to identify individual genes with confidence. One relied on the remarkable property that nucleic acid probes could be designed that would bind specifically to (hybridize with) genes based on the sequence of the nucleotides that made up the gene. A further important technology was the purification of enzymes derived from bacteria that would cleave DNA in specific places. The developers of this technique—Hamilton Smith, Daniel Nathans, and Werner Arber—received the Nobel Prize in Physiology or Medicine in 1978. These DNA cleaving enzymes are designated *restriction enzymes*. There are many different restriction enzymes, each cutting DNA in different places

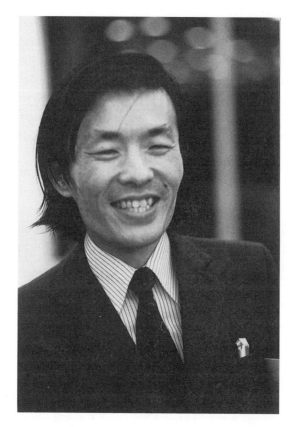

Figure 8.1. Susumu Tonegawa in the 1970s. (Courtesy of Susumu Tonegawa)

because they identify short sequences of nucleotides and then cut the DNA within the sequences they identify. These dual technologies allowed Susumu Tonegawa and his colleague Nobu Hozumi, working at the Basel Institute of Immunology in the mid-1970s, to make a breakthrough discovery that helped resolve the debate between germline and somatic mutation theory.[3]

Tonegawa (figure 8.1) was then a young scientist, born in Japan but trained in the United States. He had earned his PhD in molecular biology at the University of California, San Diego, and then worked as a postdoctoral fellow with Renato Dulbecco at the Salk Institute in La Jolla, applying molecular techniques to cells from humans and other animals, not simply to bacterial cells, as had been the dominant theme in prior years. Tonegawa had been supported by a Fulbright Award at the Salk Institute,

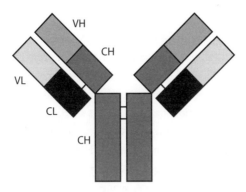

Figure 8.2. Model of an antibody molecule. The light-gray-shaded area represents the light chain variable region (VL); the darker-gray-shaded area, the heavy chain variable region (VH); the darkest-gray-shaded areas, the heavy chain constant regions (CH); and the black area, the light chain constant region (CL). The lines connecting chains represent disulfide bonds between cysteines (sulfur containing amino acids) in two adjacent chains. The "bend" in the CH chains indicates a "hinge" found in some antibody molecules that allows flexibility.

but the expiration of that award and US visa regulations required that he leave the United States. He was offered a position at the newly founded Basel Institute of Immunology, a basic research center fully funded by the pharmaceutical giant Roche. The director of the Basel Institute was Niels Jerne (whom I discussed at some length in chapter 7). Jerne proved to be a remarkable leader for the Basel Institute. His philosophy was to offer talented young scientists independence very early in their careers. This paid off beautifully in Tonegawa's case and made the Basel Institute the leading immunology center in Europe.

A little background is required to understand how Hozumi and Tonegawa's experiment resolved the controversy about how specificity was acquired. Their solution focused on the genes for BCRs/antibodies. Antibody molecules consist of two different types of protein chains that are linked to one another. One type of chain is designated H for heavy; the other, L for light (figure 8.2). There are two different classes of L chains, κ and λ. An individual antibody molecule consists of two identical H chains and two identical κ or two λ L chains.[4]

Both the H chains and L chains have portions that vary strikingly from one antibody-producing cell to another. Because of their variability, these portions have been designated V (variable) regions. The V regions contribute to the formation of the site on the antibody molecule that actually binds the antigen. For the κ and λ chains, the remainder of the chain is similar and is designated the C (constant) region.

Tonegawa and others had developed probes that would hybridize with L chain V or C regions. Another giant of this field, Phil Leder, then working at NIH, had used hybridization techniques to count the number of times a κ chain C gene was found in the genome. His research showed that there were only two or three copies of the Cκ region per genome, clearly incompatible with the germline theory, whereby each antibody L chain that could be made would have to be coded for by an "intact" L chain gene. If that were correct, then the L chain C region genes should have been present in large numbers.

One factor slowed progress in Leder's lab and the labs of other US scientists interested in molecular genetic problems. In 1975, a moratorium was agreed to that limited certain types of "recombinant DNA" experiments until more safety information could be obtained. Leder and others had to put several experiments on hold while the rules for carrying out this type of work were being formulated.

Tonegawa, in Switzerland, was free to push ahead, and he did so brilliantly. He derived a probe that would identify the V region of the κ L chain of the immunoglobulin in a particular plasmacytoma, designated MOPC321, and one that identified the κ C region, which was common to all κ chains. This allowed him and Hozumi not only to determine how many copies of the κ C region were present but more importantly to see whether these genetic elements were in the same relative position in the genome in cells that were not part of the immune system, particularly in sperm and egg cells and in antibody-producing cells.

Hozumi and Tonegawa prepared samples of DNA from MOPC321 plasmacytoma cells, representing antibody-producing cells, and from mouse embryos. Because the embryo contains no antibody-producing cells, this DNA would be drawn exclusively from nonimmune cells. Hozumi and Tonegawa cut these DNA samples with restriction enzymes so that the length of any individual segment was relatively short. They then separated these "restriction fragments" of DNA in an electrical field according to their size on a medium in which they could identify the genes they were interested in by determining whether their probes bound to them. The

Embryo   Myeloma

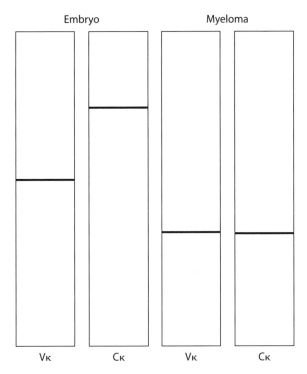

Vκ   Cκ   Vκ   Cκ

Figure 8.3. Hypothetical representation of change in relative positions of Vκ and Cκ genes in antibody-producing cells compared to those in embryo cells. DNA was isolated from mouse embryos or from a plasmacytoma (MOPC321), representing a malignant antibody-producing cell. The DNA was cut with a restriction enzyme into a large number of small fragments. The fragments were separated from one another based on their size and the fragment identified that contained the Vκ region, using a probe specific for the Vκ of the MOPC321 plasmacytoma, and the fragment containing Cκ identified by a probe for Cκ. In the embryo DNA, the MOPC321 Vκ and Cκ were on separate fragments, as seen from their different sizes (the larger fragment is closer to the "top" of the separation medium). In the DNA from the MOPC321 plasmacytoma, the MOPC321 Vκ and Cκ were on a single fragment of the same size and different from the sizes they were on in the embryo DNA.

probes had been made radioactive so that the location of given genetic sequences was indicated by the localization of radioactivity among the size-distributed set of restriction fragments (figure 8.3).

In most cell types, including embryo cells, the genes for the MOPC321 V region and the κ C region were not found on the same fragment when the

DNA was cut with a series of different enzymes. This finding indicated that the V and C genetic elements encoding the MOPC321 κ L chain were not immediately next to one another in the germline. However, when the scientists performed the same experiment using DNA prepared from the MOPC321 plasmacytoma, the genes for the Vκ and Cκ regions were located on the same fragment, indicating that in the course of the differentiation of cells to mature antibody-producing cells, a gene rearrangement process had occurred, resulting in the apposition of genes that, in nonlymphoid cells, were far apart.

The Tonegawa group and others, most notably Leder's group and the group headed by Leroy Hood at Cal Tech, followed up this breakthrough with a detailed analysis of these genetic events. The picture that has emerged is that the H and L chains are encoded separately from one another, on different chromosomes; κ and λ L chains are also separately encoded.

Taking the κ L chain as an example, its V region was actually constructed by assembling two different genetic elements designated Vκ and Jκ. In the human genome, there exist more than seventy different Vκ genetic elements and five Jκ elements. There is an enzymatic recombination "machine" that, as an example, joins one of the Vκ elements, n-1, now designated Vκn-1 (figure 8.4) to the Jκ element 3 (Jκ3) by cutting out the DNA that normally separates them. This combined Vκn-1Jκ3 element is close to the single Cκ element and, when the DNA is copied into mRNA, creates a message that specifies a κ L chain consisting of Vκn-1Jκ3Cκ. This simple strategy permits a relatively large number of distinct κ chains to be created from a limited amount of genetic information by random recombination of the Vκ and Jκ elements.

The process for H chain assembly is similar in principle but more complex. H chain V (V_H) regions are constructed from three separate genetic elements, V_H, D, and J_H. Each of these exists in the genome in multiple copies. One of the D regions rearranges to be next to one of the J_H regions, creating a DJ_H element. This recombination event is followed by a second in which one of many V_H genes rearranges to be linked to the existing DJ_H element creating a $V_H DJ_H$ element, encoding the V region of the H chain. Furthermore, there are special mechanisms to increase diversity both by imprecision at the sites of the joining of D to J_H and of V_H to DJ_H and by adding and/or removing nucleotides at the $V_H D$ and DJ_H junctions. Indeed,

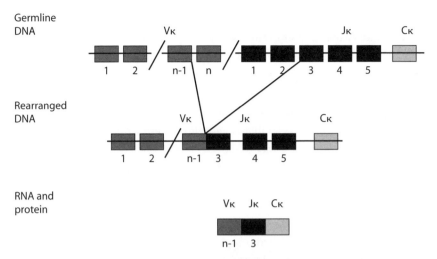

Figure 8.4. The rearrangement process through which one (Vκn−1) of many (1 through n) Vκ elements is combined with one (Jκ3) of five Jκ elements to produce a rearranged VκJκ element consisting of Vκn−1 and Jκ3. The Vκ DNA elements are rendered in grey with four indicated: 1, 2, n−1, and n. The Jκ elements are in black; all five are illustrated, and the single Cκ element is in light gray. The rearranged DNA is transcribed into an mRNA specifying a κL chain consisting of Vκn−1Jκ3Cκ.

the amount of diversity generated in this region is immense, so much so that the sequence of amino acids corresponding to the sequence of nucleotides spanning the $V_H D$ junction to the DJ_H junction can be essentially random. This region of extreme variability plays a critical role in determining the binding specificity of an antibody.[5]

Thus, taking the relatively large numbers of distinct V_H and Vκ regions that can be created by the combinatorial use of their constituent genetic elements and the enormous diversity achieved by the "random sequence generator" in the $V_H DJ_H$ junctional region, the number of individual H chains and κ chains that can be assembled is vast. The potential diversity is still further increased by the random, or at least partially random, pairing of H and L chains in individual cells.

How many different antibody molecules can be generated by this mechanism is a matter of debate, but it is surely in the millions and probably much greater. Similar mechanisms exist for the development of diverse repertoires of T-cell receptors. Thus, a substantial but not enormous amount of germline-encoded genetic information can underlie the potential to develop an essentially unlimited array of BCRs and TCRs. Of course, this means that elements of both the germline and the somatic mutation theories are correct.

The Recombination Machine

In order for the assembly of genetic elements into a V_H or V_L region to occur, there has to be a way to move the DNA encoding the distinct elements that are initially far apart into apposition with one another. This requires a mechanism to cut the DNA just "downstream" of the V element and just upstream of the D or J element to which it will be joined and then to form a joint between the cut ends.

Since DNA consists of two complementary strands, the cleavage event involves breaking both DNA strands, that is, forming double-strand breaks (DSBs). This is important because DSBs create *genome instability* with the possibility of moving (transposing) bits of DNA into sites into which they should not "go" and with subsequent risk of malignant transformation.[6] Indeed, many cancers of lymphocytes (leukemias and lymphomas) are marked by just such gene transposition, creating new genes that code for molecules that cause the formation of cancer cells. These new genes are called *oncogenes* (*onco* being derived from a combining form of the Greek noun *ónkos*, meaning mass or bulk).

A specialized enzyme system has evolved to cleave just downstream of V elements and upstream of J elements (and both upstream and downstream of D elements) and to reseal the cut ends with high efficiency so that the formation of oncogenes is a rare event. This system is dependent on two proteins, designated RAG1 and RAG2 (for recombinase activating genes 1 and 2), that recognize special DNA sequences located close to the sites that will be cleaved. The critical importance of RAG1 and RAG2 is demonstrated by the fact that if either protein is nonfunctional as a result of mutation, an affected individual fails to generate mature T or B cells and develops a severe immunodeficiency, such as David Vetter suffered (see chapter 1).

The biochemical reactions through which the cleavage and rejoining occurs has been worked out in great detail by many scientists. Just as mutations in RAG1 and RAG2 lead to severe immunodeficencies, mutations in the other proteins that are required for this recombination machine to function normally can also lead to immunodeficiencies. In the absence of the recombination machine, or when it functions abnormally, the process through which immunologic specificity is achieved is defective. Thus the immune response does not occur at all or does so only very inefficiently.

One can judge when in the developmental history of T cells and B cells they become competent to undergo the formation of BCRs or TCRs by assessing when the RAG1 and RAG2 enzymes are expressed. In general, RAG1 and RAG2 are found in precursors of B cells, in the bone marrow, and in T-cell precursors within the thymus.

The introduction of modern technologies of molecular biology and protein chemistry have combined to give us a detailed picture of how the immense amount of information required to generate an essentially unlimited array of BCR/antibody molecules and TCRs was obtained. This understanding has also taught us the root causes of certain severe immunodeficiency diseases and how many of the cancers of lymphocytes develop.

9

B Cells and T Cells Recognize Different Types of Antigens

As we have seen, antibody molecules are specific for three-dimensional structures, usually for antigenic determinants found on the surfaces of particular pathogenic microbes such as bacteria and viruses. Antibodies can also be formed against antigenic determinants on the surface of proteins, polysaccharides, or lipids. Antibodies are the products of clonal descendants of B cells. The receptors of a B cell and the antibody its descendants will make are the same, taking into account that somatic hypermutation may change antibodies as a result of mutation. The B-cell receptor, like antibody, is specific for all manner of three-dimensional structures and can bind to these on the surface of the pathogen before it has infected a cell, while it is still in the blood or in the fluid surrounding cells (extracellular fluid).

The specificity pattern of B cells makes sense in terms of the function of B cells and of the antibodies they produce. Antibodies have the job of eliminating pathogenic microbes or preventing them from infecting cells. They do this by binding directly to the infectious agent. Such binding can neutralize the pathogen by interacting with the chemical structure on the surface of the pathogen through which it would have gained entry into and thus infected a cell. In this way, the antibody blocks the infectious capacity of the pathogen; it *neutralizes* the pathogen.

But that is not the only way that antibodies can rid the body of microbes. By binding to the surface of a microbe, antibody can mark the microbe for cells that can phagocytose it (literally "eat it up") and then destroy it. These phagocytic cells are white blood cells such as *macrophages* ("big eaters") and smaller cells known as *neutrophilic granulocytes* (named because they have granules that stain neutral when researchers apply certain dyes to identify white blood cell types).

Antibodies also recruit certain chemicals in the blood that can destroy microbes by punching holes in the surface of the infectious agent. These molecules, referred to as *complement*, also have other ways of eliminating bacteria. Thus, antibodies either directly block infectious agents from entering cells by binding to them or recruit powerful "innate" defense mechanisms that can destroy these agents.

T-Cell Specificity

T cells mediate protection in entirely different ways, and the differences in their function compared to that of B cells are reflected in the specificity of their receptors. T cells do not make specific soluble products like antibodies that bind directly to the surface of infectious agents. They mediate virtually all of their functions through their interactions with other cells.

Perhaps the most "classic" of the functions of T cells is their ability to kill cells that are infected with viruses or, in certain cases, to kill tumor cells. In the case of type 1 diabetes, killer cells destroy the insulin-producing cells of the islets of Langerhans, in the pancreas. But the function for which killer cells evolved was to destroy cells that were infected with viruses or malignant by recognizing viral or tumor antigens on the surface of their "target" cells. Killer cells have a specialized mechanism through which they can punch holes in the surface of these target cells, using a molecule called *perforin*, and then inject enzymes into the cell that start a process leading to cell death.

In some cases, T cells mediate their function by increasing the capacity of other cells to destroy pathogens. For example, a T cell can recognize antigens of pathogens on the surface of macrophages and as a result produce particular cytokines, specialized molecules that increase the capacity of the macrophage to destroy the bacteria that it has ingested. Cytokines produced by T cells have many functions that can mobilize a wide range of protective functions and initiate inflammation.

T cells also act as "helper" cells, as we have seen. When a B cell has bound an antigen from a pathogen through its receptor, the B cell can display a fragment of the antigen on its surface bound to a major histocompatibility complex (MHC) molecule. The receptor of a particular type of T cell, a Tfh cell, can recognize this fragment on the B-cell surface and will bind to that B cell. Through a variety of mechanisms it then acts to strongly stimulate the B cell to make antibody.

It should be clear that if all T-cell functions require that the T cell recognize the antigenic determinant for which it is specific on the surface of another cell, then the T cell needs to avoid recognizing that antigen when it is simply in the blood or in the extracellular fluid. That would simply "distract" the T cell for no purpose. T cells have evolved a recognition specificity that is quite different from that of B cells. This recognition strategy ensures that it binds antigens only on the surface of other cells where it will then perform its effector functions.

MHC Molecules

Understanding the specificity of TCRs was one of the great accomplishments of immunological science. Reaching that understanding required the efforts of many scientists and took many twists and turns, probably because how it actually works is quite complex.

Bacteria enter cells such as macrophages or dendritic cells through a process in which they are engulfed in small, membrane-bound structures called *vacuoles*. The type of vacuole into which exogenous bacteria (or proteins) enter is referred to as an *endosome*. Endosomes and their close partners *lysosomes* contain a variety of enzymes that break down the bacterial components, including their constituent proteins, into fragments. These enzymes will chop up the proteins of a bacterium into short peptides, often consisting of a stretch of nine or ten amino acids. These cleaved products then bind to MHC molecules that have entered the endosome and the lysosome.

MHC molecules have a specialized groove that contains several deep pockets into which chemical projections of the peptides may bind. Peptides, whose structure is such that they can bind tightly into these grooves, are loaded into the complementary MHC molecule (figure 9.1). The resulting peptide-MHC complex is transported to the cell surface. This complex, consisting of an MHC molecule and a peptide derived by breakdown of a microbe or soluble protein, is the antigenic determinant actually recognized by the TCR. Different TCRs recognize different peptide-MHC complexes.

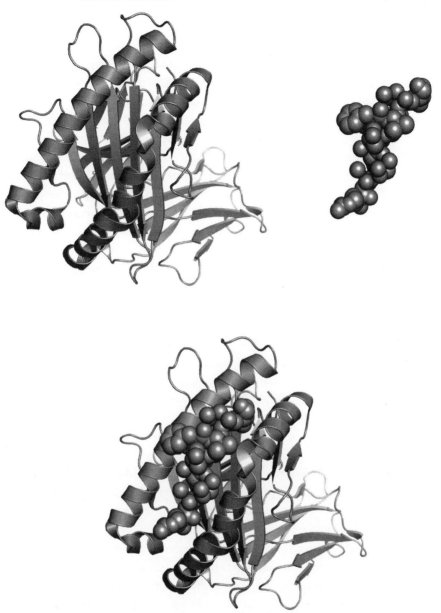

Class I MHC molecule

Peptide

Peptide-loaded class I MHC molecule

Figure 9.1. Major histocompatibility molecules bind antigen-derived peptides into a specialized "groove." The left top image represents a "ribbon" diagram of a class I MHC molecule that has not yet bound a peptide; the top right image represents a "space-filling diagram" of a peptide that is capable of being bound by that class I MHC molecule. The lower image represents the peptide bound into the groove of the MHC molecule. This conjoint peptide-MHC complex is the structural element that T-cell receptors of CD8 cells can bind. (Courtesy of Dr. David H. Margulies)

Thus, the TCR does not recognize a microbial surface protein and interact directly with that microbe. Rather, it binds to a cell surface molecular complex consisting of a peptide product, derived by enzymatic degradation of the microbe after it has entered a cell, and an MHC molecule, whose specialized groove is able to bind that peptide. This peptide-MHC complex is principally expressed on the surface of the cell that ingested the microbe and thus, of necessity, a T cell bearing a TCR specific for the peptide-MHC complex recognizes its "antigen" only on the cell surface.

This description simplifies several aspects of a more complex process. There are basically two distinct sets of MHC molecules, class I and class II, and two large families of conventional T cells, CD8 and CD4 T cells. In general, CD8 T cells recognize peptide-MHC complexes containing class I molecules while CD4 T cells recognize peptide-MHC molecules containing class II molecules. Furthermore, the CD4 T cells recognize peptide-MHC complexes in which the peptide is generally derived from a microbe that has been imported into the cell, for example by phagocytosis. By contrast, CD8 T cells recognize peptide-MHC complexes in which the peptide is derived from a product of the cell itself, such as when a virus has infected the cell and its products are made by the cell or, in the case of the recognition of a peptide derived from a tumor antigen, when the tumor antigen is a product of the malignant cell.

Thus, CD4 T cells are adapted to recognize and respond to exogenous products imported into a cell although they also can recognize cells in which bacteria may live within the endosome and produce their products there. These products are then degraded and loaded into class II MHC molecules. The bacteria that cause tuberculosis, *Mycobacteria tuberculosis*, for example, live within endosomes.

CD8 T cells are adapted to recognize and destroy tumor cells and virus-infected cells. In the case of a virus-infected cell, it would be ideal if the cell killing event occurred before the infected cell makes sufficient virus to infect another cell. Newly synthesized viral proteins (or tumor-specific proteins) are broken down to peptides within the cytoplasm, often in an assemblage of proteins known as a *proteasome*. These peptides are then transported into the structures where class I MHC molecules are being produced and are loaded into the binding groove of the molecules. Having completed the loading process, the complexes are transported to the cell surface where they can be recognized by TCRs on CD8 T cells.

As we have gained a fuller understanding of the diversity of lymphocytes and of their distinctive functions, it has become clear that the immune system has evolved in such a way as to match the cell's function and immune-recognition mechanisms. This alignment is yet another example of the highly sophisticated nature of the modern immune system.

10

My Foray into the Specificity Problem

Antibodies and B-cell receptors recognize three-dimensional structures, and antibodies have evolved to neutralize or eliminate pathogens through their capacity to bind to molecules on the surface of these pathogens. By contrast, T-cell receptors recognize a complex consisting of a major histocompatibility complex molecule and an antigen-derived peptide that is bound into a specialized groove in the MHC molecule. Thus, the type of specificity shown by B cells and T cells is very different. So how did we learn this?

My research project in Baruj Benacerraf's laboratory when I arrived there in 1964 was to study precisely this question. I was to measure the specificity of T and B cells from guinea pigs immunized with well-defined antigens and test whether their pattern of specificity was the same or different. I had to do the research using methods that would allow me to obtain quantitative data, not simply to make a qualitative statement that they seemed different.

To study the specificity of antibody, I immunized guinea pigs with a very simple antigen, a polymer made up of many copies of a single amino acid, L-lysine. The *L* refers to the fact that most amino acids are optical isomers (remember the distinct forms of tartaric acid) that rotate polarized light either clockwise (*levo* or L) or counterclockwise (*dextro* or D). All naturally occurring amino acids are L in type. To the polymer of L-lysine, designated poly-L-lysine (PLL), we attached a small number of organic molecules. They were conjugated to only a few of the lysines in the polymer. The organic molecules we used were benzene rings with nitro groups at particular positions on the ring (2,4-dinitrophenyl [DNP]).

The PLL carrier (recall from chapter 6 that when a protein is bound to a small molecule, that molecule is called a *hapten* and the protein a *carrier*) was essential for immunogenicity, but a guinea pig immunized with DNP-PLL did not respond to PLL alone; indeed, the bulk of the antibodies produced were directed against the DNP group. My first task therefore was to make precise measurements of the specificity of these anti-DNP antibodies that appeared when the guinea pig was immunized and to estimate the proportion of the energy that binding to the simple compound DNP-L-lysine (DNP conjugated to a single lysine) contributed to its binding to the DNP-PLL immunogen.

We needed several steps to make these measurements. Of course, the first was to prepare the DNP-PLL, taking care to keep the number of DNP groups on a single PLL molecule low. If I placed too many groups on a PLL molecule, I would alter its structure as a whole, with the possibility of confusing the results. Once I had prepared DNP-PLL, I immunized the guinea pigs with this compound.

However, it was not simply a matter of injecting the DNP-PLL into the guinea pigs. In order to get a robust antibody response, an *adjuvant* has to be injected with the antigen. Understanding how adjuvants work can help unlock key principles governing immune responses. Children who receive the classical DPT (diphtheria, pertussis, and tetanus) vaccine are given a compound, alum (potassium aluminum sulfate), with the vaccine. Alum acts as an adjuvant, resulting in marked enhancement of their response to the vaccine. In experimental animals, more potent adjuvants than are safe for humans can be used. The adjuvant I used was complete Freund's adjuvant, named for Jules Freund, the scientist who had developed it. Complete Freund's adjuvant consists of killed tuberculosis bacteria in an oil-in-water emulsion. (More on adjuvants in chapter 21.)

After several weeks, the guinea pigs had made sufficient amounts of anti-DNP antibodies that I could purify them from the blood. I won't go through the purification procedure, but suffice it to say I could obtain pure antibodies all of which were able to interact with DNP-L-lysine. Now the problem was how to measure the "specificity" of these antibodies.

But what precisely do we mean by specificity? Answering this requires understanding some simple chemistry. When two molecules are mixed together, they may bind to one another if the arrangements of their atoms are such that there is some "complementarity" between them. The simplest analogies would be the "binding" of a hand in a glove or a key in a lock, although chemical complementarity is often quite different from these obvious examples. The "tightness" of the interaction between two molecules can be thought of as the amount of energy that would need to be applied to force the interacting molecules apart after they had bound to one another. The energy necessary to disrupt their bond is related to the equilibrium constant (K) of the binding of the two compounds. In principle (but not always in practice), the equilibrium constant is quite easy to determine.

If molecule a and molecule b interact to form the new molecule ab, we would say:

$$a+b \rightarrow ab$$

When the reaction is complete, K is calculated by dividing the concentration of the resultant molecule ($[ab]$) (i.e., in molecules per volume) by the product of the concentrations of the reactants ($[a]$ and $[b]$) at equilibrium.

So the formula for K is very simple:

$$K = [ab] / [a] * [b]$$

K then can be converted to the energy needed to disrupt ab to its constituents by the following equation:

$$Energy = R * T * lnK$$

in which Energy is actually the change in energy since it is the amount added to disrupt the bond, R is a constant (called the gas constant), T is temperature (measured in relationship to absolute zero), and lnK is the natural logarithm of the equilibrium constant, which we have just determined.

It could be said that an antibody is specific for that molecule for which it has the highest energy of binding. If one wished to do the measurements, one could determine a "landscape of specificity" by measuring the energy of binding of the antibody to a whole series of related molecules.

So my project was to measure the equilibrium constant of the binding of the purified antibody for the simplest representation of DNP, in this case DNP bound to a single lysine (DNP-L-lysine), and to compare it to the equilibrium constant of its binding to the immunizing compound, DNP bound to PLL. I was fortunate that a procedure had just been developed, called *fluorescence quenching analysis*, that made it easy to make these measurements. The result was that around 90 percent of the energy of binding to DNP-PLL of the anti-DNP antibody produced in response to immunization with DNP-PLL could be accounted for by its binding to DNP-L-lysine. That is, the specificity of the antibody, and thus the BCR on the precursor of the antibody-producing cells, was very much concentrated in its specificity for the hapten.

Now the second part of my project was to ask about the T-cell receptor. At that time, we did not know what the TCR was chemically, so I couldn't do an experiment that paralleled our antibody experiment. But I could do a functional experiment. I used a slightly different model from what I had used to measure antibody specificity. Again, I immunized guinea pigs with a DNP-carrier conjugate, although rather than using DNP-PLL, as I had for determining antibody specificity, I used a conjugate of DNP to a guinea pig protein, guinea pig albumin. The reason for choosing guinea pig albumin as the carrier is that guinea pigs are tolerant to it and thus do not make an immune response specific for unmodified guinea pig albumin. The capacity to elicit a response is dependent on the conjugation of the DNP group to the guinea pig albumin, so I didn't have to worry about the response to unmodified guinea pig albumin.

Once the immunization was complete, I needed a quantitative test to measure the specificity of the T cells. While I couldn't make the precise energy measurements I had done for antibody, I devised a test through which I could quantitatively compare the capacity of a DNP–guinea pig albumin conjugate to elicit a T-cell response to that of a DNP conjugate of some other protein, such as cow albumin. I could also ask whether DNP-L-lysine elicited a response.

The test was as follows: I prepared sterile suspensions of lymphocytes from the lymph nodes of the immunized guinea pigs and placed them in tissue culture. It had just been shown that adding the immunizing antigen to a lymphocyte culture would make some of the T cells in the culture divide, presumably those T cells that were specific for the test antigen. I could easily measure the cell division rate because when cells divide they have to make new DNA. Nucleotides, the molecules that make up the DNA, have to be incorporated into the cells and then into the DNA. One of these nucleotides, thymidine, was easily available in radioactive form, so the measurement was simply how much radioactive thymidine was taken up and incorporated into the DNA.

The results were unequivocal. The immunizing antigen, DNP–guinea pig albumin, caused massive T-cell division, as shown by the uptake of large amounts of radioactive thymidine into the DNA. Other proteins to which DNP was conjugated, including the DNP–cow albumin conjugate, elicited virtually no uptake of thymidine, even at very high concentrations. Nor did DNP-L-lysine cause any DNA synthesis.

I could clearly say that when immunizing with a hapten-carrier conjugate, the antibody response was largely hapten-specific; the carrier made only a very modest contribution to specificity. By contrast, the T-cell response required that both the hapten and the carrier be the same. Although shown in this one system, this concept is a general one and applies widely.

My experiment in the Benacerraf lab was just the first step on the road to understanding that B cells and T cells deal with different antigenic universes, with the BCR being specific for three-dimensional structures as they exist in solution while the TCR recognizes a MHC-peptide complex.

Obviously, it is a long way from showing the "carrier specificity" of T-cell responses to recognizing that what the T cells "see" is an antigen-derived peptide loaded into an MHC molecule. But along that winding path was a key discovery my colleagues and I made.

11

Genes and Immune Responses

During my time working with Baruj Benacerraf, I had made great strides in understanding the specificity of T cells and of B cells, using antibodies as a surrogate for the B-cell receptors. But by 1967, it had become clear that staying at New York University was not an option for me.

Neither was it an option for Benacerraf, it turned out. Baruj was by then recognized as one of the leading immunologists of the day. Once it was known he was available, many offers came in. The most attractive was chief of the Laboratory of Immunology (LI) in the National Institute of Allergy and Infectious Diseases (NIAID) at the National Institutes of Health. Baruj was attracted to LI because the resources available were far greater than he had at NYU and thus he could develop a more integrated research program. But he had a second reason. The NIH offered Baruj access to inbred guinea pigs.

Baruj had demonstrated that the allelic form of a particular gene an experimental animal possessed controlled that animal's capacity to make an immune response to very simple antigens. When he immunized a population of guinea pigs obtained from a local supplier with DNP-PLL, the molecule I used in the experiment detailed in chapter 10, only about 40 percent of the guinea pigs would make an immune response. The remaining 60 percent were nonresponders. He had done careful breeding between responders and nonresponders and had concluded that the difference between them could be accounted for by differences in a single gene that he referred to as an *immune response* (Ir) gene. Responsiveness to DNP-PLL showed simple Mendelian inheritance.

Baruj had done a great deal of work aiming to understand the nature of this genetic control, but he was hampered by the variability in the frequency of responders and nonresponders in any group of guinea pigs. Furthermore, because they were not inbred, it was difficult to transfer cells from one guinea pig to another in order to understand what cells controlled the ability to respond. Two inbred strains of guinea pigs did exist, however, strain 2 and strain 13, and both were available at NIH in large numbers but virtually nowhere else in the world. Fortunately, strain 2 guinea pigs could respond to DNP-PLL and strain 13 guinea pigs could not.

Baruj invited Ira Green and me to join him in the LI, which we were both happy to do. I continued my interest in the specificity of T-cell responses and worked closely with Ira on the mechanism underlying the genetic control of immune responses. During Baruj's first year at NIH, however, he was offered the chairmanship of the Department of Pathology at Harvard Medical School, the position he'd hoped for when he first decided to leave NYU. He accepted and left NIH in 1970.

Although Baruj asked me to join him at Harvard, I was reluctant to do so for several reasons. Marilyn and I were happy in Maryland, and our boys, Jonathan and Matthew, were well placed in school. I also was concerned that were I to move with Baruj for a second time, I would be making an announcement of dependency when what I really wanted to do was to establish that I could be successful as an independent scientist. That would be hard to do if I continued to work in a setting where my former mentor remained my "boss."

Marilyn and I decided that we wouldn't move to Boston. But who would replace Baruj as LI laboratory chief? John Seal, the scientific director of NIAID, was charged with recruiting a new leader for LI. He announced that Robert Schwartz, an eminent hematologist from Tufts University School of Medicine, would take the position. While I believed that Dr. Schwartz would be a good leader, I thought I ought to see if there were other opportunities. I was pleased to receive several attractive offers, including one at the Washington University School of Medicine in St. Louis.

While Marilyn and I were mulling over this job offer, the announcement was made that Bob Schwartz had reconsidered and was not coming to NIH, so the lab chief position was open again. John Seal then decided that he would choose an NIH scientist as chief. There were several individuals more senior than I who surely could have been considered. However, Ira Green strongly encouraged me to apply. This allowed Baruj to throw his influence behind my candidacy, and I was offered the position, which I was delighted to accept. So at age thirty-four, I moved into my new office, on the eleventh floor of the NIH Clinical Center, as the youngest lab chief on the NIH campus.

At LI we conducted a set of experiments that I believe were instrumental in understanding how Ir genes worked. What we found played an important role in clarifying what the TCR recognized. The experiments were actually very simple. As I pointed out, there were two inbred strains of guinea pigs available at NIH, strain 2 and strain 13. These inbred strains of guinea pigs had been developed many years earlier at the US Department of Agriculture and included many more strains but in the course of a move to a new facility, the guinea pigs were transported in an open wagon and exposed to a rainstorm. As a result, all but two strains (2 and 13) were lost. Fortunately, the remaining two strains were sufficient for our work.

Strain 2 guinea pigs could respond to DNP-PLL and to a series of related compounds including a random co-polymer of two amino acids, glutamic acid and lysine (GL) and to a DNP conjugate of GL (DNP-GL), whereas strain 13 guinea pigs could not. Ira and Baruj had shown that there were a set of antigens to which strain 13 guinea pigs could respond but to which strain 2 guinea pigs could not. The "index" antigen was the random co-polymer of glutamic acid and tyrosine (GT). The offspring of the mating of the two inbred strains, (2x13)F1 guinea pigs, could respond to both sets of antigens.

In 1969, after we had moved from NYU to NIH, the one other scientist who was seriously interested in Ir gene control of immune responsiveness, Hugh McDevitt at Stanford University, made a crucial discovery. With his colleague Allen Chinitz, McDevitt mapped the location in inbred mice of the Ir gene controlling responsiveness to a co-polymer made up of tyrosine, glutamic acid, alanine, and lysine to the major histocompatibility complex of genes. This linkage of an Ir gene and MHC genes opened the door to a true understanding of TCR specificity.

MHC genes were so named because differences in this set of genes were the major determinants of whether skin and tissue grafts from a donor to a recipient would be rapidly rejected or not. The MHC gene products were accordingly called *transplantation antigens*. The finding that the genes that determined the capacity of mice to respond to simple antigens were linked to the genes for transplantation antigens was stunning. Ira and Baruj, working with Leonard Ellman and William Martin, rapidly confirmed the linkage of MHC genes and Ir genes in guinea pigs. It would later be proved that Ir genes and MHC-encoded genes for transplantation antigens were identical.

With the knowledge of the linkage of Ir genes to the MHC, Ira Green and Ethan Shevach, a young postdoctoral fellow, prepared antibodies that were specific for the MHC gene products of strain 2 guinea pigs and antibodies specific for the MHC gene products of strain 13 guinea pigs. Ethan, Ira, and I then did what I believe to be a critical experiment.

We immunized (2x13)F1 guinea pigs with a mixture of DNP-GL and GT in complete Freund's adjuvant. The F1 guinea pigs responded to both antigens. We prepared lymphocytes from immunized F1 guinea pigs and tested their responsiveness in tissue culture to both antigens, using the radioactive thymidine uptake assay I had developed at NYU. We observed that the F1 lymphocytes responded to DNP-GL and to GT. The F1 cells also responded to a component of complete Freund's adjuvant known as the purified protein derivative of tuberculin (PPD) (figure 11.1). These responses required that a population of F1 cells be present that had the property of adhering to tissue culture dishes. These cells functioned as *antigen-presenting cells* (APC). At the time, we thought the cells that mediated APC function were macrophages, but actually the most potent APCs in this population were dendritic cells.

We now had primed F1 T cells that in the presence of F1 APC could respond to an antigen to which strain 2 but not strain 13 cells could respond (DNP-GL), to an antigen that strain 13 but not strain 2 cells could respond (GT), and to an antigen to which both strain 2 and strain 13 cells could respond (PPD). We also had antibodies specific for strain 2 MHC proteins and for strain 13 MHC proteins, and we knew that the Ir genes mapped to the genetic region that encoded the strain 2 and strain 13 MHCs. Furthermore, the antibodies were mainly specific for class II MHC molecules, and while they did not bind to the guinea pig T lymphocytes, they strongly bound the guinea pig APCs.

The critical question was, would the anti-2 and the anti-13 antibodies, binding principally to the APCs, not the lymphocytes, have any effect on the response of the F1 T cells to DNP-GL, GT, or PPD? The answer was clear. The anti-2 antibodies completely inhibited the response of the F1

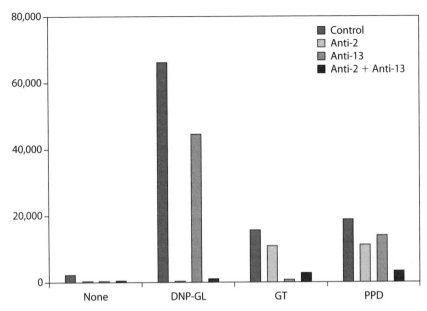

Figure 11.1. Anti–class II MHC antibodies specifically inhibit Ir gene-controlled T cell proliferation. Responses are measured by DNA synthesis shown as uptake of radioactive thymidine (0 to 80,000 cpm). The T cells are stimulated with no antigen (none) or by DNP-GL, GT, or PPD. The effect of adding no antibody (control) or anti-2, anti-13, or anti-2 plus anti-13 antibodies is illustrated in the bar graph. (Adapted from *Journal of Experimental Medicine* 136 [1972]: 1207–21, table 4)

lymphocytes to DNP-GL, had little or no effect on their response to GT, and had only a modest effect on their response to PPD. The anti-13 antibodies completely inhibited the response of the F1 T cells to GT but not to DNP-GL and had an only modest effect of their response to PPD. A mixture of the two antibodies completely blocked responses to all three antigens.

Since the class II MHC molecules were expressed on the APC and not the T cells, this result implied that the APCs were the critical cells in which the Ir genes operated. Furthermore, if the blockade of the class II molecule by the antibody blocked antigen-presenting function, the implication was that the class II molecule mediated the antigen presentation and that the allelic form of the class II molecules associated with responder status was essential for a response to occur.

Ethan Shevach teamed up with a colleague from an adjoining laboratory, Alan Rosenthal, to do a related experiment, again using F1 cells from donors primed to DNP-GL, GT, and complete Freund's adjuvant. They placed the lymphocytes from the immunized donors in tissue culture and varied the source of the APC. What they found was that APC from a strain 2 donor would stimulate a response to DNP-GL but not GT while APC from a strain 13 donor would stimulate a response to GT but not DNP-GL. Either APC could induce a response to PPD. This result strengthened the contention that Ir genes operated in the antigen-presenting cell, not the T cell, and that the APCs with the responder form of the MHC could successfully present the antigen, whereas cells with the nonresponder form of the MHC could not.

These experiments were persuasive and pointed the way to the solution that the TCR recognized a peptide-MHC complex on the APC and that Ir genes or MHC genes determined whether such presentation could occur. The implication was that the responder form of the Ir gene encoded a class II (or class I) MHC molecule that could bind the peptide while the nonresponder form encoded an MHC molecule that could not bind the peptide.

A disadvantage of our experiments was that they were performed in guinea pigs. We knew far less about the guinea pig MHC than that of the mouse, and we had only two inbred strains of guinea pigs whereas there were many mouse inbred strains. The mapping of the mouse MHC had been done with great precision; that of the guinea pig was still at a very early stage. There was no doubt that the mouse would be a far better experimental model in which to study this linkage of Ir gene function and MHC gene products. Indeed, a year later, Rolf Zinkernagel and Peter Doherty, studying the MHC requirements for CD8 T-cell killing of cells infected with lymphocytic choriomeningitis virus, established that such killing required that the MHC type of the responding T cell and of the target cell be the same, confirming the concept of "histocompatibility restriction" that we had demonstrated and doing so in a system in which their mapping of the MHC genes and the genes controlling the capacity of the cells to mediate cytotoxicity was unambiguous. Zinkernagel and Doherty received the 1996 Nobel Prize in Physiology or Medicine for their work.

Ron Schwartz, a new postdoc in my research group, repeated and then extended our work studying Ir gene control of antigen-stimulated T-cell proliferation using inbred mice. To do this, he had to solve what had been a technological barrier; it had been very difficult to carry out the antigen-stimulated T-cell proliferation assays using mouse cells. Ron solved this problem and was then able to carry out experiments that established that the Ir genes controlling CD4 T-cell responses were class II MHC genes.

The ultimate proof came somewhat later, when another of my postdoctoral fellows, Laurie Glimcher, showed that a point mutation in a class II MHC molecule, resulting in the change of only a single amino acid, altered the Ir gene-controlled antigen-presentation function of APC expressing this mutant class II MHC molecule. Laurie went on to a truly distinguished career and is now dean of the Weill-Cornell Medical College. In chapter 22, I describe an elegant experiment she carried out illuminating the pathogenesis of inflammatory bowel disease.

As we were finishing this work, Emil Unanue, whom Baruj had recruited to Harvard Medical School from the Scripps Research Institute in California, showed that purified class II MHC molecules could directly bind peptides. Furthermore, he demonstrated that responder forms of class II MHC molecules could bind peptides that would elicit a response in these mice while the nonresponder forms of class II MHC molecules would fail to bind the same peptides. This discovery completed the journey. Ir gene function consisted in the capacity of class II MHC molecules on APC being able to bind peptide in a conformation such that they could be recognized by the TCR.

Thus, the Ir gene story starts with the simple observation that some animals can respond to a simple antigen and some cannot. It ends with an entirely unprecedented recognition event in which the capacity of simple molecules to elicit a T-cell immune response is determined by whether the MHC molecules expressed on that animal's APCs can or cannot bind a peptide derived from the immunogen.

One set of observations that indicates that these observations with simple antigens in experimental animals are almost certainly important in human immune responses comes from a genetic analysis of susceptibility to human autoimmune diseases. To try to understand what genes predispose to the autoimmune disorders, researchers have used various approaches to determine the relative susceptibility of individuals who have different allelic forms of different genes. In general, the results have been disappointing. No single common allelic form of any gene seems to contribute a great deal to risk. But there is one glaring exception. That exception is the MHC genes. The form of an MHC gene an individual possesses may increase his or her risk to develop an autoimmune disease strikingly. One of the most dramatic examples is ankylosing spondylitis, a chronic inflammatory disease of the axial skeleton with variable involvement of peripheral joints. More than 90 percent of individuals diagnosed with ankylosing spondylitis have the HLA type B27; the frequency of B27 in the general population is about 8 percent. Another striking example is that almost 50 percent of Caucasian children who develop type 1 diabetes have a single allelic form of a class II MHC gene. These observations imply that the principles that underlie antigen-presentation of simple antigens in experimental animals underlie whether an individual will make an immune response that causes the development of autoimmune diseases.

12

The Laboratory of Immunology and

the T-Cell Receptor

One of the great problems of immunology into the early 1980s was determining the biochemical nature of the T-cell receptor. Once the clonal selection theory had been accepted, it was clear that the B-cell receptor must be an immunoglobulin molecule, specialized to reside in the cell membrane. This was established experimentally by David Naor and Dov Sulitzeanu from the Hebrew University Hadassah Medical Center in Jerusalem and by Gordon Ada of the Australian National University in Canberra. They independently showed that B cells specific for a particular antigen could bind that antigen to their surface using their membrane immunoglobulin. I had heard both teams present their striking findings at the first international meeting I attended, in Slapy, Czechoslovakia, in 1969, and was enormously impressed.

On my return to NIH, I set up a major research project on that problem with Joseph Davie, an extremely talented postdoctoral fellow. Joe had earned a PhD in bacteriology from Indiana University and an MD from the Washington University School of Medicine. He had spent time in the laboratory headed by Richard Krause at the Rockefeller University. After leaving my lab, Joe had a brilliant career, serving as chairman of the Department of Microbiology at Washington University School of Medicine, then as chief scientific officer at the pharmaceutical company G. D. Searle, and finally as senior vice-president for research at Biogen, a leading biotech firm.

Joe and I showed how the affinity of the B-cell receptor increased over the interval since immunization, which was a prediction of the effect of somatic hypermutation on the increase in antibody affinity with time. We demonstrated that in tolerant animals, the cells that escaped tolerance had lower affinity receptors than did the cells of nontolerant animals, a finding clearly predicted by the clonal selection theory. We also showed that each B cell had but a single type of receptor, as the theory also predicted.

The study of the BCR was proceeding well during the 1970s, but we were making little progress in understanding the TCR. The big stumbling block was that we had no a priori knowledge of what the T-cell receptor was. However, by 1982, several groups had amassed biochemical evidence for the existence of a T-cell surface protein that appeared to vary from one T-cell clone to another, strongly suggesting that it was the TCR.

The overarching goal was to identify the gene or genes that coded for the TCR. That would allow an understanding of the chemical nature of the TCR, as well as of how its diversity was attained. A major breakthrough resulting in the identification of the gene for one of the chains of the TCR came from a set of elegant experiments Mark Davis did at LI.

Mark had worked with me as a postdoctoral fellow but then carried out this remarkable piece of work independently. Mark had earned his PhD at the California Institute of Technology under Leroy Hood. Hood was engaged in building on Susumu Tonegawa and Nobu Hozumi's experiment that showed how genetic mechanisms underlay the creation of the great diversity seen in BCRs (see chapter 8). Mark and another student were the leaders of the Hood group's program in working out the genetic mechanisms involved in immunoglobulin gene rearrangement and class switching. Mark came to visit LI because he felt that he needed to learn immunology. Although he had accomplished so much, he still thought that his knowledge of immunology was deficient. His view was that the best place to learn immunology would be in LI as my postdoc. I was honored, although I was not as convinced as Mark was about my standing among immunologists. Nonetheless, I was delighted to welcome him to LI.

We discussed various experiments he might do. Taking advantage of his extensive knowledge of molecular genetic techniques, we decided that he would try to understand the difference between the patterns of genes that B cells and T cells transcribed into messenger RNA. To put this a little less ambitiously, we would attempt to determine what percent of genes that were expressed by T and B cells were shared and what percent of the expressed genes were different. Today, this would be a simple experiment that any graduate student could do, but in 1980 it was a challenge to even the most able molecular geneticist.

Mark used a technique known as cDNA subtraction, which relied on the fact that the opposite strands of DNA from a gene bind to each other with great specificity and very tightly. This property could be taken advantage of to establish which expressed genes were shared and which were different. Mark reached the conclusion that the B and T cells differed in their expression of about 2 percent of their genes. He identified some interesting genes in which they differed, and that allowed him to clone the gene for a particular class II MHC chain that had not been previously identified.

Based on his success in using cDNA subtraction, Mark developed a strategy he believed would allow him to clone the gene or genes that encoded the TCR. It was clear to all of us in LI that Mark was a scientist of immense ability and great creativity. With the strong support of all the LI senior staff, I decided that Mark should be set up in an independent lab so he could try out his strategy. We found a module that we could make available. One of my other postdoctoral fellows, David Cohen, and one of Ron Schwartz's postdocs, Steve Hedrick, volunteered to join Mark, and a technician, Ellen Nielsen, was assigned to him.

Mark's idea was that the TCR gene should have three critical properties. It should be expressed in T cells and not B cells; the protein it encoded should be expressed on the cell surface; and it should consist of genetic elements that would be far apart in non-T cells but would be close together in T cells. He had already worked out the techniques to purify T-cell–specific genes during his postdoctoral work with me. It was known that messenger RNAs that encoded proteins expressed on the cell surface were usually associated with ribosomes (the protein manufacturing organelles of the cell) that were bound to membranes. Mark and his group found ten genes that met these two criteria and then analyzed all ten to determine whether any were located on different DNA fragments, produced by digestion with restriction enzymes, in T cells and non-T cells. They found that one of the ten genes showed changes between T cells and non-T cells consistent with a rearrangement process like the one Hozumi and Tonegawa had demonstrated from the genes for the κ L chain of immunoglobulins. The gene Mark identified was sequenced. It was clearly different from the membrane immunoglobulin that was the receptor of the B cell, yet it was a member of the same structural family, and the rearrangements it went through were reminiscent of those of B-cell immunoglobulin. Mark and his colleagues designated the gene that they had cloned as the gene encoding the β chain of the TCR.

What was so remarkable was that the whole process was achieved in an eleven-month period by a small group of extremely talented young scientists who worked very hard. Furthermore, at the time, this was probably the single most competitive area of immunology. Mark and his group had succeeded in the face of great odds by the force of creativity, elegant technology, hard work, and excellent colleagues. I emphasize that this was the independent work of Mark's small group. Neither I nor any of my other senior LI colleagues were co-authors of the two papers describing this research, but we were all excited by the great accomplishment.

Needless to say, I did my utmost to persuade Mark to stay at NIH as a principal investigator, but it was not to be. He accepted an extremely attractive offer from Stanford University, where he remains a distinguished professor. Although Mark has had many triumphs at Stanford, he has in recent years devoted himself to the effort to move the focus of the best immunology research from mouse experiments to work on human cells and, where possible, to use human disease as a laboratory to understand fundamental mechanisms of immunology. I discuss this approach in chapter 32.

III THE SECOND LAW

Tolerance

13

What Is Tolerance?

Recall the young girl who came to the emergency room in diabetic coma because her own killer T cells had destroyed the β cells of her islets of Langerhans. Those killer cells had recognized and responded to an antigen expressed by her islet cells. Normally, such responses to one's own cells either do not occur or are effectively controlled through a series of biological processes. These processes collectively lead to a state described as *immunological tolerance*.

The evolutionary pressure that led to individual B cells and T cells having only one or possibly two receptors per cell was to avoid, as much as possible, destructive self-reactivity. Avoidance of self-reactivity is of such importance that several distinct mechanisms have developed to prevent responses of this type from occurring or, where they cannot be prevented, to limit any damage they may cause.

Elimination of potentially self-reactive cells as they develop, often referred to as *clonal deletion*, is one of the most important tolerance mechanisms. As we have seen, T cells or B cells sometimes acquire a self-reactive receptor through the essentially random genetic processes that underlie receptor formation. The principle of clonal deletion is that the cells with self-reactive receptors are eliminated as a result of contact with that self-antigen at particular times during development. That is, the developing cell responds to contact with antigen in a fundamentally different manner from the way the mature cell does.

The concept that antigenic experience during immaturity leads to tolerance had its beginnings in a beautiful set of observations made in the 1940s by Ray Owen, then a postdoctoral fellow in the immunogenetics laboratory at the University of Wisconsin. Owen was a Wisconsin farm boy who grew up during the depression years. He lived on his parents' farm and commuted the eight miles from home to high school and, later, to Carroll College in Waukesha, each day doing farm chores in the mornings and evenings. His obvious talents had attracted the attention of his teachers, and they encouraged him to think beyond the farm life that he had anticipated.

After completing his undergraduate degree, Owen went to Madison to do his PhD work in genetics at the University of Wisconsin. His thesis there concerned the developmental biology of hybrids between birds of different species. He completed his PhD in 1941 and joined a laboratory that studied the inheritance of blood groups in cattle.

At the time, there was considerable interest in determining cattle blood groups, both for their importance in illuminating mammalian genetics and as a way to determine paternity in cattle breeding. The immunogenetics laboratory was supported by dairy cattle associations. The laboratory had developed many antibodies to multiple cattle blood group antigens and had analyzed their mode of inheritance. Based on his analysis of blood group antigens, Owen observed that "there was something funny about twin calves."[1] When he tested the blood groups of brothers and sisters of the same parents, they were rarely alike, but when he examined twins, 90 percent of the time they had identical blood groups even though they were generally fraternal twins (half were male-female pairs). The explanation for this "funny" behavior came to Owen as a result of receiving blood samples from "an interesting pair of twins that had been born a year or so before" at the Blakeford Farms in Queenstown, Maryland.

The mother was a Guernsey cow that had been mated with a purebred Guernsey bull. Later that same day, a Hereford bull had broken into the pasture and mated with the same Guernsey cow. When the resulting twins were born, it was clear they had different fathers; one had the appearance of a purebred Guernsey, the other of a Hereford-Guernsey hybrid. Owen asked for blood samples from the three parents and was able to show that the half-sibling twins had identical blood groups but that the blood groups inherited from the Hereford bull and those from the Guernsey bull were on *different* red blood cells in each of the twins.

It was known that in the great majority of cattle twins, connections between the fetal blood vessels occurred, allowing for in utero exchange of blood-forming cells between the twins. Owen knew that had blood cells of non-twin half-siblings been exchanged as adults, the cells would have been rejected. He also knew that the cattle red blood cells did not survive more than 120 days. Since the calves were over a year old when he received their blood for analysis, the animals must have been actively producing red blood cells of both types, implying that blood stem cells must have been exchanged between the calves in utero and were functioning in the half-sibling twins.

Owen quickly reached the conclusion that the exchange of blood cells between fetal calves allowed each twin to *tolerate* the blood cells and the blood stem cells of the other twin rather than to reject those cells, as would have occurred had blood stem cells from one mature cow been transfused into another. The presence of both sets of blood cells in both twins implied that experience with genetically foreign substances at a particular stage of development resulted in the failure of the individual to make an immune response against those substances at that time and prevented them from making a response against them even when the animals were adults and thus competent to make effective immune responses against other antigens.[2]

Owen published his work in 1945 in *Science*, a leading scientific journal then just as it is today, so these observations were clearly in a prominent place in the scientific literature. Probably on the basis of this pathbreaking observation, Owen was recruited to join the Biology Division of the California Institute of Technology, where he spent the rest of his academic career.

Owen's work was insightful and his conclusions prescient. But his efforts to extend this work to a system in which he could initiate and control experiments, rather than rely on the chance events that would bring appropriate samples to him, were not successful. It remained for another team to take up this effort in a more tractable experimental system. Peter Medawar and his colleagues Rupert Billingham and Leslie Brent, in the Department of Zoology of University College London (UCL), showed that they could reproduce and extend Owen's findings in inbred mice by transferring tissue from mice of one inbred strain to fetal mice of another inbred strain.

Peter Medawar was born in Petropolis, Brazil. He was educated at Oxford and during World War II was asked to investigate the problem of skin grafting, which was an urgent matter because so many pilots were badly burned and in desperate need of grafts. Medawar showed that skin from an unrelated donor was virtually always rejected and that a second graft from the same donor was rejected even more quickly, strongly implying that rejection was an immunological phenomenon. After the war, he returned to Oxford as a fellow of one of the major colleges. In this role, he tutored Av Mitchison, whose work I describe in chapter 3 and whom Medawar influenced greatly.[3]

Medawar went on to a distinguished career, winning a Nobel Prize and becoming director of the National Institute of Medical Research in Mill Hill, London. I had the privilege of meeting him when I worked in Av Mitchison's lab for a few months in the spring of 1968. Medawar suffered a stroke in 1969, and although he continued to write and lecture, the stroke was a disabling event. I recall that he had been invited to give a major lecture at the Smithsonian Institution in Washington, DC, which Marilyn and I attended. He had his carefully prepared text in front of him, but in the course of the lecture, the pages became scrambled and he found it hard to understand what had happened. His wife, sitting in the front row, put the pages back in order and Medawar, drawing on a reserve of grace, said to her and the audience, "I see what you mean by page seven coming after page six," after which all was well.

By 1951, Medawar had moved to London to become the Jodrell Professor of Zoology at UCL, and it was there he and his brilliant team carried out a series of remarkable experiments on skin graft rejection and on the induction of a tolerant state that would allow the acceptance of foreign skin grafts. Medawar was aware of Ray Owen's work and cites Owen's *Science* paper in his 1960 Nobel Prize lecture.

The UCL group had a great advantage in understanding the mechanism of the tolerant state that Owen had observed. Using inbred mice, Medawar and his colleagues could actually do planned experiments rather than relying on the chance events in which cattle twins of different parentage were born. The UCL scientists injected tissue from inbred mice of strain A into fetal mice of a different inbred strain, CBA, and showed that the recipient CBA mice as adults would accept a skin graft from an A donor but not from a different donor. CBA mice that had not received A tissue in utero or as neonates rejected A strain skin grafts when they were implanted into them as adults, in accord with Medawar's observations on human skin grafts in his work during the war years. These experiments and others being done at about the same time, particularly by Milan Hašek in Czechoslovakia using chickens, clearly showed that tolerance could be induced if antigens were introduced into very young animals.

But was it the immaturity of the animal that made its immune system susceptible to the induction of tolerance on antigen exposure, or was it exposing immature *cells* to antigen that was responsible? This is an important distinction because lymphocytes are continuously developing from precursor cells, especially during the young adult period. All of these cells go through a development process so that they must move through an "immature" state even if they are in a mature animal. We now know that it is not the immaturity of the animal that is critical for the induction of the form of tolerance observed by Owen, Hašek, and Billingham, Brent, and Medawar but rather the "immaturity" of the developing lymphocyte when it encounters antigen that is critical to the development of the tolerant state. In an immature animal, the vast majority of all the lymphocytes are in an immature state, of course.

A sidelight to this discussion concerns two Nobel Prizes, one for tolerance, awarded in 1960 to Medawar and Burnet (figure 13.1), and one "for theories concerning the specificity in development and control of the immune system" given to Niels Jerne in 1984. The 1960 prize for tolerance to Medawar was well deserved but for Burnet is rather problematic. In his Nobel lecture, Burnet says, "My part in the discovery of acquired immunological tolerance was a very minor one—it was the formulation of a hypothesis that called for experiment." Indeed, Burnet's Nobel lecture is an exposition of the clonal selection theory, for which he clearly deserved a Nobel Prize. His prediction of tolerance was published in 1949, four years after Owen's report of induced tolerance in cattle twins in *Science*. My view is that the proper pairing in 1960 would have been Owen and Medawar.

In 1984, when the prize was awarded to Niels Jerne, Burnet was still alive, as was David Talmage. Jerne had published the first paper reintroducing the notion of selection, "The Natural-Selection Theory of Antibody Formation," which, as I discussed, lacks the critical concept that the selectable element was a cell and that specificities were distributed one to each cell. Indeed, Jonathan Uhr, an eminent immunologist who wrote a commentary on the Nobel Prize in the journal *Science* in 1984, emphasized

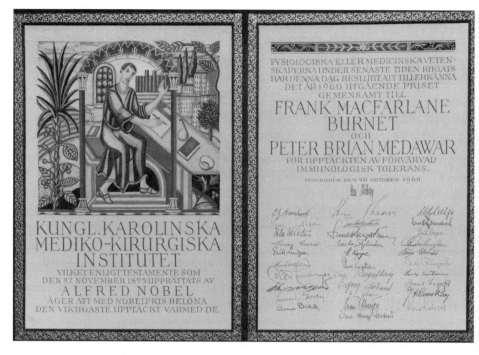

Figure 13.1. 1960 Nobel diploma for Macfarlane Burnet and Peter Medawar. (Courtesy of the Walter and Eliza Hall Institute of Medical Research and the Nobel Foundation. Copyright © The Nobel Foundation 1960, Artist: Bertha Svensson-Piehl)

Jerne's role in reawakening the idea of selection but said, "The particulars of Jerne's hypothesis needed correction, however. Burnet exploited this selective concept and properly suggested that the selection process takes place between antigen and clones of lymphocytes, each one of which produces antibody of a single specificity."[4] Talmage and Burnet conceived of clonal selection, and Burnet made it the mission of his life to persuade the scientific community of its power. Clearly, the 1984 Nobel Prize would have more appropriately gone to Burnet and Talmage.

What are we to conclude? Prize committees don't always get it right, although they try their best, and the verdict of history is a better test of the importance of one's contributions.

Regardless of Nobel accolades, what mattered most for the development of immunology was a striking pair of biological experiments—one an observation of a virtual accident, the other carefully planned and carried out. Together, they showed us that the encounter of lymphocytes with antigens for which their receptors are specific during a period of immaturity leads to the failure of the immune system of the individual animal in which the encounter has occurred to respond to that antigen when it is administered during maturity. But what is the mechanism underlying this "immaturity tolerance"? It is to this issue that we now turn our attention.

14

How Does Tolerance Develop?

Clonal selection theory provides a powerful way to account for immunological memory through the cellular response to initial encounter with antigen. Cells that respond in that initial encounter increase their numbers dramatically. Thus, secondary stimulation causes a much more vigorous response than does primary stimulation, in part because there are many more antigen-specific cells available to respond. But cells that have undergone a primary response not only increase their numbers but also undergo certain changes so that their subsequent responses are both greater in magnitude and different in type. That an initial stimulation causes the responding cells to change their characteristics is an important concept. It is a general feature of lymphocytes and makes it possible for them to be highly functional effector cells, capable of making responses appropriate to the infectious threat that led to their expansion and differentiation.

Encounter and Response

A corollary to enhanced responsiveness as a result of initial encounter with an antigen is diminished responsiveness as a result of such contact. Recall the experiments in cattle twins and inbred mice exposed to foreign tissue during fetal life described in the previous chapter. In these cases, immaturity of the immune cell rather than of the animal as a whole determined whether an encounter with antigen will induce tolerance rather than immunity.

To be more precise, the encounter of a population of specific T or B cells with the antigen for which their receptors are specific (often referred to as their *cognate* antigen) during particular developmental stages may lead to diminished responsiveness of those cells or even to their death. If all the cells in a population that are specific for a given antigen are eliminated as a result of contact with that antigen, the cell population can be said to be no longer capable of responding to that antigen; rather, it is tolerant of that antigen. Such cellular elimination tolerance, or clonal deletion, is a central mechanism for the death of self-specific T and B cells during the development of T cells and B cells. Basically, cells encountering their cognate antigens under conditions of cellular immaturity respond to that antigen challenge by undergoing a process described as *programmed cell death*; fundamentally, the antigen encounter drives the cells to commit suicide.

The implication of this process is that all developing B and T cells would be subject to a "filter" that leads to their elimination if they are specific for any antigen they encounter during development. Thus, endogenous antigens present in the same site as the developing cells should cause the elimination of cells specific for such antigens. In consequence, a substantial proportion of T or B lymphocytes specific for self-antigens should be clonally deleted.

One problem is that antigens only expressed in specific tissues in the periphery (in the pancreas or thyroid, for example) might not be available at the sites where the lymphocytes are developing. Such lymphocytes therefore would only "see" these self-antigens after they had passed through the developmental window in which contact with antigen would cause elimination. This can happen with insulin, made by the β cells of the islets of Langerhans. In these cases, we might anticipate that T cells and B cells capable of responding to insulin would not be removed by the clonal elimination process.

T-Cell Development

At least in the case of developing T cells, however, a mechanism has evolved to deal with this potential problem. First, let's review the steps in the development of T cells. T cells arise from specialized precursor cells that are found in the bone marrow. These cells traffic through the blood and enter the thymus. They go through several developmental steps, each occurring in a particular microenvironment within the thymus. As a result of these differentiation steps, the precursor cells develop into a set of thymocytes that express T-cell receptors on their surface. The most immature of these TCR-expressing thymocytes are found within a region of the thymus called the cortex. In the cortex, thymocytes encounter an unusual selection process requiring that they recognize, with some degree of affinity, self-peptide-self-MHC molecules expressed on a particular set of cortical thymocytes designated *cortical thymic epithelial cells* (cTECs). Cells that do not recognize self-peptide-self-MHC molecules on cTECs fail to survive, so what emerges from this first selection process are cells that are capable of recognizing self-MHC molecules. These cells, referred to as *positively selected* cells, then migrate from the cortex of the thymus to a new environment, called the thymic medulla.

In the medulla, those developing thymocytes whose TCRs *strongly* interact with self-peptide-self-MHC molecules on the surface of medullary thymic epithelial cells (mTECs) are eliminated by a specialized cell death process known as *apoptosis* (from the Greek for "dropping off"). The eliminated cells are said to have been *negatively selected*. This process constitutes the deletional tolerance step for T cells. However, does this mean that cells specific for a self-peptide-self-MHC complex in which the self-peptide is derived from a protein made by specialized cells in peripheral tissues survive and that such cells could constitute a major threat when they reach the periphery?

The mTECs that present self-peptide-self-MHC complexes have an unusual feature. They synthesize many proteins that we normally think of as only made in specialized tissues in the periphery, such as insulin. Thus, they can eliminate many of the T cells specific for these peptide-MHC complexes. In order to express these proteins, the mTECs rely on a molecule called AIRE (autoimmune regulator). AIRE regulates the expression of genes that encode proteins principally made in specialized tissues. Thus, through this process of negative selection, the medulla of the thymus acts as a filter to remove cells with a high degree of reactivity to self-antigens, even to self-antigens that are normally expressed only in specialized locations.

The importance of the expression of AIRE-controlled proteins in the mTECs of the thymic medulla can be judged from the consequences of mutations in the gene encoding AIRE. Humans who do not produce AIRE because of such mutations have a disease called *autoimmune polyendocrinopathy candidiasis ectodermal dystrophy* (APECED). People who suffer from APECED develop autoimmune responses to many tissues, particularly to endocrine organs such as the β cells of the pancreas, the thyroid, and the adrenal and parathyroid glands. If not recognized and treated appropriately, APECED can be fatal.

Once T cells leave the thymic medulla, they travel to the secondary lymphoid organs (the thymus is a primary lymphoid organ), such as the lymph nodes and the spleen. They are now regarded as mature but naïve, which means they have not yet encountered and responded to their cognate foreign antigens. There are situations even for such cells in which antigen encounter will lead to tolerance rather than immunity. However, the predominant mechanism that operates on mature T cells to prevent them from mediating autoimmune responses is immunological suppression, and that process is mediated by the action of a specialized population of T cells designated regulatory T cells or Tregs.

15

Regulatory T Cells and the Prevention of Autoimmunity

In a 2002 paper,[1] R. S. Wildin, S. Smyk-Pearson, and A. H. Filipovich describe a young boy who shortly after birth developed a middle-ear infection, then diarrhea; by six weeks of age the baby was in diabetic coma. While in the hospital being treated for type 1 diabetes, he developed pneumonia due to choriomeningitis virus, a herpes-type virus that rarely causes disease in normal people. The child's continuing diarrhea was diagnosed as inflammatory bowel disease. At about the age of one, he was found to have massive enlargement of his lymph nodes and spleen to the extent that he had difficulty breathing because his tonsils and adenoids were obstructing his airways.

Before the age of two, he developed an infection with Epstein-Barr virus. This is the virus the causes infectious mononucleosis, usually in much older children and teenagers. At two, he was diagnosed with hypothyroidism (diminished function of the thyroid often due to autoimmunity) and at two and a half, he developed autoimmune hemolytic anemia, in which antibodies to his red blood cells caused them to burst.

That he survived until the age of five, when his case was reported, is a testimony to the skill of his physicians and modern medicine. The litany of horrific problems that this poor child experienced was shown to be due to his failure to develop Tregs. He was born with a mutation in an X-chromosomal gene that coded for the protein Foxp3, which is essential for the function of Tregs. The disease resulting from the lack of Foxp3 function is called immunodysregulation, polyendocrinopathy, enteropathy, X linked (IPEX), and it illustrates the central role that Tregs play in protecting us from autoimmune disease.

The idea that the response of T cells and B cells might be controlled by other lymphocyte populations, initially designated *suppressor T cells*, dates back to the late 1960s. However, methodological difficulties with those early studies led to great skepticism about whether suppressor T cells actually existed, and consequently the suppressor T-cell field went into a decline, only to be rescued by a series of experiments conducted by Shimon Sakaguchi, initially when he was working in the laboratory of Professor Y. Nishizuka in Nagoya, Japan, and then in his own laboratory.

Nishizuka had observed that if a mouse had its thymus removed between two and four days of age, it later developed severe autoimmune responses involving the ovary (oophoritis), the stomach (gastritis), the thyroid (thyroiditis), or the testes (orchitis). Crucially, if the thymus was removed earlier (on the day of birth) or later than day four, these abnormalities did not occur.

Three-Day Thymectomy

Sakaguchi showed that if he took T cells from these "three-day thymectomized" mice that were undergoing autoimmune responses and injected them into mice that lacked their own T and B cells, the donor cells would cause the appearance in the recipient of the autoimmune response seen in the donor. This experiment established that the autoimmunity was due to T lymphocytes that were primed in the three-day thymectomized donor. But what was truly remarkable was that if he injected T cells from normal donors of the same strain into the three-day thymectomized mice within two weeks of thymectomy, the autoimmune responses were prevented. This experiment implied that there was a population of cells in normal mice that could prevent or reverse the T-cell-mediated tissue auto-inflammation and that these cells were absent in three-day-thymectomized mice.

Working in Oxford in parallel with Sakaguchi's research in Japan, Fiona Powrie and Don Mason showed a similar phenomenon. They were interested in the properties of T-cell populations transferred into rats that lacked any T cells of their own. The rats they worked with are called nude rats. Nude rats bear a mutation that causes abnormalities in hair development but, more importantly for our purposes, leads to the failure of the thymus to form. These athymic rats thus fail to develop a T-cell immune system.

What Powrie and Mason observed was that if they removed a particular set of T cells (those characterized by having very small amounts of a cell surface marker designated CD45RC) from T-cell populations derived from normal rats and transferred the remaining T cells into nude rats, the recipients would develop a wide range of autoimmune disorders including thyroiditis and type 1 diabetes. They also showed that co-injecting the CD45RC^{low} cells would prevent these autoimmune diseases.

Both the Sakaguchi and Powrie and Mason experiments implied that some cells that had emigrated from the thymus to the secondary lymphoid organs could cause a wide range of autoimmune responses. Such responses indicated that clonal deletion tolerance had not been complete. But another population of T cells must have existed that kept these potentially autoreactive T cells in check. Because the term *suppressor T cells* had fallen into such disrepute, the designation *regulatory T cells* (Tregs) was applied to these cells. Tregs are now one of the most intensively studied of lymphocyte populations.

CD25, Tregs, Foxp3, and IPEX

Sakaguchi continued to work on defining the properties of the Tregs that both revealed important features of their biology and aided in their identification. He showed that Tregs expressed on their surface large amounts of one component of the receptor for an important cytokine. Cytokines, as we have seen, are products of T cells through which they mediate their function. One, interferon-gamma, enhances the capacity of macrophages to destroy bacteria that they have ingested, for example. But there are many different cytokines, each mediating a group of critical functions. Particularly critical is the cytokine *interleukin-2* (IL-2).

IL-2 regulates the growth and survival of lymphocytes. Tregs are especially dependent on IL-2, and they express on their surface a large number of molecules known as CD25, which are part of the cell surface receptor through which IL-2 acts. In general, one can identify Tregs in mice and in people because these of the high levels of CD25 they express.

The real breakthrough in studying Tregs came from the analysis of humans and mice that suffered from IPEX. As we learned from the case of the severely sick boy discussed at the beginning of this chapter, IPEX is a genetically determined autoimmune disease of boys that results in severe enlargement of lymphoid organs, type 1 diabetes, and inflammation of other endocrine organs, severe eczema, and inflammatory bowel disease. Unless treated with bone marrow transplantation, affected individuals often die during childhood. A similar genetically determined disease was noted in a strain of mice, referred to as *scurfy mice*, so named because they presented with scaly or dried skin. These mice displayed immune abnormalities that resembled those of IPEX patients and which, like IPEX, was caused by the mutation of a gene on the X-chromosome.

In 2001, Fred Ramsdell and his colleagues in Seattle showed that both IPEX and the scurfy abnormality could be accounted for by mutations in the X-chromosomal gene *Foxp3*, which worked by regulating expression of other genes. An important component of the process of gene expression is the *transcribing* of genes (copying DNA into messenger RNA) and molecules that control this process are designated *transcription factors*. The protein encoded by the *Foxp3* gene is a transcription factor also designated Foxp3 (genes are designated in italics; proteins in roman type).

But at first researchers were unable to establish the exact relationship between Foxp3 and the severe autoimmunity seen in IPEX and scurfy mice. Two years later, three research groups, headed by Sakaguchi, by Ramsdell, and by Alexander Rudensky, simultaneously discovered that Foxp3 was essential for the development of Tregs and that, in normal individuals, Foxp3 was mainly expressed in Tregs. When Foxp3 is absent, Tregs completely fail to develop, whereas in the other situations, such as the three-day thymectomy, there is only partial diminution in numbers of Tregs. Even more than previous studies, this finding of the difficulties faced in the absence of Foxp3 established how critical Tregs are to avoiding autoimmunity.

Clearly, the absence of Tregs leads to a truly devastating autoimmune state. The severe abnormalities of IPEX patients and scurfy mice indicate that while clonal deletion in the thymus is surely important, it alone will not prevent the immune system from targeting the host. Indeed, enough potentially autoreactive T cells escape clonal deletion that, unless Tregs are present, these cells cause fatal autoimmune diseases.

How Do Tregs Work?

The mechanism of operation of Tregs remains a controversial subject. Tregs appear to have many modes of action through which they control the function of other lymphocytes. My own interpretation is that

Tregs evolved to control highly self-reactive conventional T cells that had escaped negative selection in the thymus and that the primary function of Tregs was to prevent the activation of these self-reactive T cells even when they were stimulated by their cognate self-antigen. However, once Tregs had evolved, they probably took on additional functions that are now of great importance. Other scientists, however, maintain different opinions on the central role of Tregs.

Positive and Negative Selection

To explain this process, let's begin with reviewing the role of the thymus. As described in chapter 14, the thymus is a filter that selects cells that are potentially able to respond to foreign antigens but eliminates those cells that react strongly to self-antigens. Once thymocytes express TCRs, they are subject to selection processes. The first type of selection occurs in the thymic cortex. In this initial process, survival of TCR-expressing thymocytes requires that they recognize self-peptide-MHC complexes expressed on cTECs. If they fail to interact with these peptide-MHC complexes, they will die through the process of apoptosis.

Thymocytes are selected for survival because they can bind to a *self*-peptide-MHC complex even though their eventual function will depend on their ability to recognize a *foreign*-peptide-MHC complex. There has been much discussion of why this is so. In my view, no wholly convincing explanation has been advanced. Nonetheless, it is the case that this process of *positive selection* in the thymic cortex leads to the elimination of a set of thymocytes that do not recognize self-peptide-MHC complexes and presumably would fail to recognize any foreign-peptide-MHC complex. Thus, thymocytes that have "failed" positive selection can be regarded as essentially useless to the individual.

Thymocytes that "passed" positive selection next move to the thymic medulla where they undergo negative selection. Those cells whose TCRs bind to a self-peptide-MHC complex very tightly (i.e., with high affinity) are eliminated, again by being induced to undergo apoptotic cell death. However, some cells that interact with a self-peptide-MHC complex with a relatively high affinity, rather than undergoing apoptotic cell death, are stimulated to develop into Tregs.

Thus, Tregs that develop within the thymus are selected because they can recognize self-peptide-MHC complexes with reasonably high affinity.

This specificity is critical to their function to limit auto-reactive responses on the part of the other populations of T cells, often designated *conventional T cells* to distinguish them from Tregs.

Tregs and Dendritic Cells

As we have seen, the cognate antigen of a T cell is a peptide-MHC complex. This complex can in principle be formed on the surface of any cell that expresses class I MHC molecules (for CD8 T cells) or class II MHC molecule (for CD4 T cells). However, although such recognition events do occur on many cell types, the events that are most important for the priming of a naïve CD4 or CD8 T cell mainly occur when the T cell recognizes its cognate peptide-MHC complex on the surface of a dendritic cell (DC). Dendritic cells are excellent at presenting peptide-MHC complexes to T cells, and they also express other molecules that play cooperating roles in T-cell activation, through a process often referred to as *co-stimulation.*

Dendritic cells take up foreign antigens or microorganisms and break down their constituents into peptides of limited length. These peptides are loaded into the specialized grooves of MHC molecules and then transported to the cell surface where T cells that have cognate TCRs can recognize them.

What determines whether this interaction leads to the activation of the T cell? Surely, the strength of interaction of the TCRs of the conventional T cells with the expressed peptide-MHC complex on the surface of the antigen-presenting DC is one factor. But a "strong" interaction does not appear to be enough. The DC is usually found in a "resting" state in which it expresses relatively small numbers of MHC molecules and relatively few co-stimulatory molecules. Among the most important of these molecules are CD80 and CD86, which engage a critical co-stimulatory pathway mediated by the T cell surface molecule designated CD28. Thus, antigen presentation by resting dendritic cells often leads to little or no response on the part of CD4 or CD8 T cells that have TCRs that can recognize the expressed peptide-MHC complexes because of the relatively small numbers of these complexes and the poor expression of co-stimulatory molecules on these cells.

The key then as to what determines the effectiveness of the interaction of conventional T cells with a DC that expresses its cognate peptide-MHC complex is the activation state of the DC. But what determines dendritic cell activation? My own view is as follows. When a dendritic cell presents a peptide-MHC complex to a T cell whose TCR is specific for that complex, the T cell expresses a cell surface molecule that binds to and activates the DC (figure 15.1A; DC is "on"). Tregs prevent this activation process, keeping the DC in a resting state and thus unable to activate the T cell (Figure 15.1B; DC is "off"). For the Treg to do this, it must also recognize a peptide-MHC complex on the very same DC, thus bringing the Treg to the same DC to which the conventional T cell has bound or will bind.

This inhibitory effect of Tregs on DC activation can be overcome. Dendritic cells engaging both Tregs and conventional T cells can be activated through a process of pathogen sensing or danger sensing. Recall that pathogen-associated molecular patterns (PAMPs) have the capacity to activate the immune system. PAMPs can act directly on DCs to activate them, even if the DC is being restrained by a Treg, or they can act on another cell that then will communicate with the DC through the production of a factor often referred to as a *danger signal*, which can activate the DC. Thus, a DC that undergoes strong pathogen sensing or danger sensing will become activated even if it is being suppressed by a Treg (figure 15.1C; DC is "on").

What is the outcome of such a system? First, it means that the simple interaction of self-reactive T cells with DCs will generally not lead to T-cell activation since Tregs will also interact with those DCs and prevent their activation. Second, it means that DCs expressing a foreign peptide-MHC complex will also not activate T cells with cognate TCRs because the dendritic cells will be prevented from becoming activated by the action of Tregs. Here is where adjuvants come into play.

Adjuvants mimic the effect of pathogens or danger signals and allow dendritic cells to become activated even in the presence of Tregs. However, this function carries with it a risk. In the course of an infection or when antigens and adjuvants are administered, DCs presenting self-peptide-MHC complexes may become activated and, in consequence, conventional T cells that recognize self-peptide-MHC complexes with reasonably high affinity may respond. This scenario almost certainly does occur, although there are backup mechanisms that limit the extent of such self-reactivity. In general, the self-reactive cell response terminates when the pathogen is eliminated or when the adjuvant effect ends. Tregs again control the state of activation of the dendritic cells and the autologous response terminates.

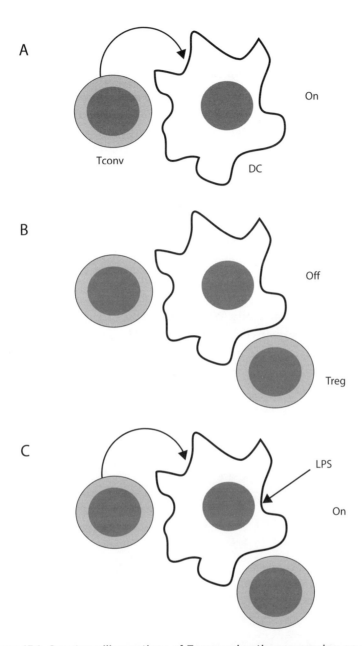

Figure 15.1. Countervailing actions of Tregs and pathogen sensing on dendritic cells (DC) and on DC-mediated T-cell activation. (A) In the absence of Tregs and pathogen sensing, conventional (Tconv) CD4 T cells recognize antigen presented by a DC and activate that DC, leading to reciprocal activation of the Tconv cells. (B) In the presence of regulatory T (Treg) cells, DCs activation is prevented and Tconv cells remain quiescent. (C) LPS is recognized by a pathogen sensor (TLR4), thus activating DC and Tconv cells even in the presence of Treg cells.

Tregs have additional functions that control the action of conventional T cells not only by blocking their initial priming but also by controlling the function of these cells in the tissues where they mediate their damaging effects. While these functions are very important, I believe they are secondary in significance to the effect of Tregs in controlling initial priming by preventing the activation of dendritic cells.

Tregs and pathogen-sensing oppose functions as part of a finely tuned balance. This balance helps explain why adjuvants are needed to induce robust immune responses.

Tolerance is a central aspect of the immune response. If tolerance fails to develop normally, the individual pays an enormous penalty. Violating the second law of immunology carries a great cost. Even the partial loss of the clonal elimination pathway, seen in patients with AIRE deficiency, causes severe autoimmunity. What would be the case if all clonal deletion failed can only be guessed, but surely it would be devastating. But despite the necessity of clonal deletion, there are sufficient numbers of potentially self-reactive cells that escape to the periphery that without the action of Tregs, survival is unlikely.

IV THE THIRD LAW

Appropriateness

Different Structures, Different Functions

Different pathogens have very different lifestyles and inhabit distinct niches within the body. For an immune response to be effective, it must be "appropriate" to the pathogen. Different kinds of antibodies mediate different types of protection.

Antibodies were the first components of the immune system recognized. They neutralize toxins and directly block the capacity of microbes to enter cells. As we have seen, they have other functions as well, such as binding to pathogens and marking them for phagocytosis (eating) by macrophages or neutrophilic granulocytes. Antibody-bound bacteria can also be destroyed through the action of the complement system.

Are all of these functions mediated by a single type of antibody, or are there different types of antibodies for different functions? We need to be careful here. Different *types* of antibodies should not be confused with antibodies of different binding specificity. Types are different in the means through which antibodies that have bound to an antigen lead to its neutralization or elimination. That is, antibodies have different functions.

Let's first take a closer look at the structure of antibodies. Recall the experiment done by Arne Tiselius and Elvin Kabat in Sweden in which they showed that purified antibodies were globular proteins that had a relative mobility in an electrical field arbitrarily called "gamma" (in comparison to alpha and beta proteins that migrated more rapidly). Thus, antibodies were termed *gamma globulins*. Tiselius and Kabat estimated the molecular weight of the antibodies at about 150,000 daltons.[1] The designation *gamma globulin* has now been replaced with the term *immunoglobulins* (Igs). I also pointed out that antibodies consist of a unit (sometimes more than one unit) comprised of two H chains and two L chains and that there are two distinct types of L chains, κ and λ.

Let's examine some of the experiments through which we learned of the structure of antibodies. Two scientists made the major contributions to deciphering their structure: Rodney Porter at the National Institute for Medical Research in London and Gerald Edelman at the Rockefeller University in New York.

Porter prepared purified rabbit gamma globulin and subjected it to digestion with the enzyme papain.[2] He found that papain digestion of the purified gamma globulin molecule gave rise to two distinct fragments, both with a molecular weight of about one-third that of the starting protein (figure 16.1). One of the fragments formed crystals but did not have the capacity to bind to antigens while the second fragment, which did not crystallize, retained the antigen-binding activity of the untreated antibody. Porter named these fragments Fab (antigen-binding fragment) and Fc (crystallizable fragment) but how they were oriented in the intact molecule was not clear nor was the function mediated by the Fc portion of the antibody.

Gerald Edelman used a different strategy. It was known that intact proteins often consist of more than one polypeptide chain. These chains are often linked to one another by bonds between the amino acid cysteine in each of the chains. Cysteine is a sulfur-containing amino acid, and the bonds that form between different chains of a protein are usually between the sulfur atoms of cysteines in the two chains (hence "disulfide bonds"). Therefore, one could get information about the chain structure of a protein by breaking these disulfide bonds through a process called *reduction*. To do this completely, the molecule had to be unfolded. Edelman dissolved the protein in a solution of urea to disrupt many of the interactions between different amino acids that hold the protein in a particular shape. When Edelman dissolved antibodies in urea and subjected them to conditions that cleaved the disulfide bonds, he obtained two types of products, one of a molecular weight of about 50,000 daltons and one of a molecular weight of about 25,000 daltons. These proved to be the H and L chains.

What was the relationship between Porter's Fab and Fc fragments and Edelman's H and L chains? Through continued work by both the Porter and Edelman groups and by several others, it became clear that Porter's Fab consisted of Edelman's L chain linked through a disulfide bond to a

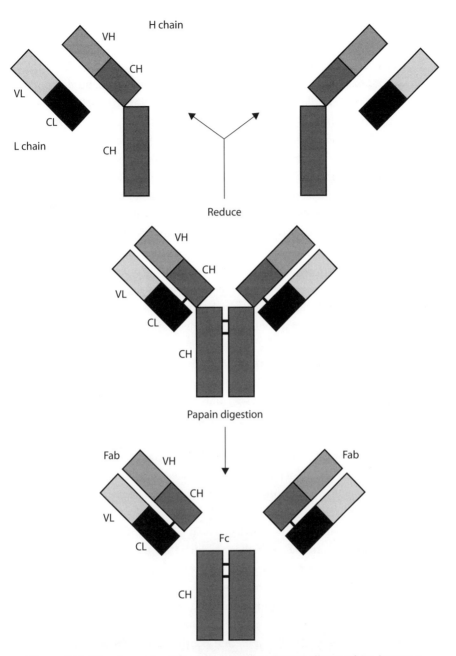

Figure 16.1. Structure of antibody molecules. Porter digested an immuno-globulin molecule with the enzyme papain, yielding one Fc fragment and two Fab fragments each of around 50,000 daltons. Edelman treated an im-munoglobulin molecule by reduction (breaking disulfide bonds) and dena-turation, blocking interactions between immunoglobulin chains, yielding products (heavy chains) of 50,000 dalton and (light chains) of 25,000 dal-ton molecular weight, respectively.

portion of Edelman's H chain and that the Fc consisted of two copies of the remainder of Edelman's H chain, linked to each other by disulfide bonds (see figure 16.1). While the L chain linked to a portion of the H chain was the antigen-combining component of antibody, the Fc portion proved to contain the region of the antibody molecule that mediates its functions.

This analysis of the structure of immunoglobulin earned Porter and Edelman the 1972 Nobel Prize in Physiology or Medicine. When it was possible to determine the actual amino acid sequences of all the components, it became clear that antibodies differed from one another in sequence. As expected from the genetic structure, discussed in chapter 8 with Hozumi and Tonegawa's experiment, the differences in the protein sequence were concentrated in certain regions of the antibody molecule. The L chains could be described as consisting of two domains, each of about 110 amino acids in length. The L chain domain closer to the "tip" of the antibody varied markedly from antibody preparation to antibody preparation and accordingly was called the *variable region of the light chain* (V_L). The remainder of the L chain was constant in structure and thus designated the *constant region of the light chain* (C_L).[3]

The structure of the H chain was more complicated. The portion of the H chain in Porter's Fab fragment at the tip of the molecule also contained a variable region designated V_H. However, the remainder of the H chain consists, in most cases, of three constant (C_H) domains, each domain again being about 110 amino acids in length. Between the first and second C_H domains, there is often a hinge region that provides flexibility to the antibody molecule.

The C_H domains of H chains come in different forms that convey different functions to the antibodies of which they are a component. These different H chains are designated in lower case Greek letters and the antibody molecules they are part of have the homologous upper case Roman letter. Thus, the μH chain is part of an antibody designated IgM. The other classes are γ, IgG (of which humans have four subclasses); α, IgA; ε, IgE; and δ, IgD. IgM expressed as a membrane protein, together with IgD, is the main receptor of naïve B cells. IgM, as a secreted protein, is the first type of antibody made. IgM antibodies consist of five copies of the basic antibody unit of two H and two L chains; IgM antibodies are very efficient in binding to and neutralizing pathogens and can engage the complement system.

IgG in humans has four subtypes: IgG1, IgG2, IgG3, and IgG4. They vary but overlap in their functions. For example, IgG1 is far better than IgG2 in sensitizing bacteria for phagocytosis by macrophages and neutrophils. It is also far superior to IgG2 in crossing the placenta and thus equipping the neonate with a sampling of his or her mother's antibodies to protect against infections. IgG3 is the best activator of complement.

IgA mainly acts at mucosal surfaces such as in the intestine, lung, and urogenital tract. Its main function is to prevent bacteria at these surfaces from entering the tissues of the body. IgA often consists of a multiple of two antibody units. IgE is the principal mediator of allergic inflammatory symptoms.

The initial antibody produced is IgM. The other classes of antibodies (except for IgD) are produced by a complex process in which the gene encoding the heavy chain V region (the V_H genetic element) moves from its initial position next to the gene encoding the μ C_H domains (the $C\mu$ gene) to a new position, next to a different C_H region (e.g., $C\gamma_1$). This process is called antibody class switching. (I discuss it in greater detail in chapter 27.)

Class switching occurs in the germinal center, a specialized structure in the lymph nodes and the spleen. It depends on a special population of T cells called *T follicular helper* (Tfh) cells. Tfh cells are also present in the germinal center where they mediate their function in helping B cells to produce antibody and to undergo the processes of class switching and somatic hypermutation.

Which of the different classes of antibody are produced (that is, to which class the B cell switches) is determined by the properties of the Tfh cell that is in the germinal center with the antigen-specific B cell. The cytokine or cytokines the Tfh cells produce determine the class of Ig to which the switch occurs. This phenomenon has been studied in greater detail in the mouse than the human. For example, switching to mouse IgG1 and to mouse IgE is controlled by the cytokine IL-4. Switching to mouse IgG2a (mouse and human subclass designations are different) is determined by interferon-gamma (IFNγ). Switching to IgA is controlled by yet another cytokine, TGFβ. The type of differentiated Tfh cell determines the nature of the antibody that is made and in turn the protective value of that antibody or, more properly, determines that the antibody made is appropriate to the type of infection that induced the response. Thus, the type of Tfh cell that appears in an immune response determines that the type of antibody produced will be appropriate to the threat.

Scientists now have techniques that allow them to determine the precise location of atoms within the antibody molecule. The most widely used technique is X-ray crystallography, which depends on the refraction of X-rays by the individual atoms of the antibody (or indeed of any protein). Through complex mathematical reconstruction, very accurate models of the positions of all the atoms in an antibody molecule have been obtained.

Monoclonal Antibodies

Though not directly related to appropriateness, the subject of *monoclonal antibodies* has assumed great consequence in treatment of many diseases and needs to be considered. As I discussed in chapter 1, monoclonal antibodies to the cytokine TNFα have revolutionized the treatment of rheumatoid arthritis and Crohn's disease. But what is a monoclonal antibody?

Recall from the discussion of clonal selection that each naïve lymphocyte has a unique set of receptors. When an individual is immunized, those naïve cells whose receptors can bind an antigenic determinant on the immunogen sufficiently well will be stimulated, and they will expand in number and differentiate. The B cells among them will develop into antibody-producing cells. As it is likely that many different B cells recognize the immunizing antigen but do so in different ways, the antibody response will be heterogeneous; it will be made of a collection of unique antibodies produced by the descendants of each responding B cell. Some of these antibodies will have very favorable properties, others will not.

Georges Köhler and Cesar Milstein, at the Laboratory of Molecular Biology in Cambridge, UK, recognized that if they could immortalize each of these different antibody-producing cells, they could then choose the one whose antibodies had the most useful properties, expand it, and obtain an essentially unlimited amount of those antibodies. That is essentially what they did.

The technique involves immunizing an animal with an immunogen. In the case of the monoclonal anti-TNFα antibody used to treat rheumatoid arthritis and Crohn's disease, the immunogen was TNFα. This particular procedure was actually done by Jan Vilcek at the NYU School of Medicine to produce the monoclonal antibody that was the basis of the treatment of rheumatoid arthritis and Crohn's disease. Once the immunized animal had developed a robust antibody response, its lymphocytes were purified and fused with cells of a cultured tumor line that had been derived from an antibody-producing cell in which the genes for antibodies had been lost. The fused cells, called *hybridomas* (a hybrid of a single antibody-producing cell and a single cell derived from the tumor cell line), had the growth properties of the tumor cell and the antibody-producing property of the antibody-producing cells. The hybridomas were then grown in tissue culture, one hybridoma to a culture well. The antibodies produced by each hybridoma were then tested for the properties desired, in this case, the ability to block the action of TNFα very efficiently. Those with the best properties were selected for expansion and further study. The hybridoma that had the best properties was then chosen to be propagated. Because a single antibody-producing cell was fused to form the hybridoma, the antibodies produced by the hybridoma would be identical to one another and could be obtained in essentially unlimited amounts.

If the antibody-producing cell fused to form the hybridoma was derived from a mouse, the product of the hybridoma would be a mouse antibody. Such an antibody could be used to treat humans, but since it was a foreign (mouse) protein, the human recipient might soon make an antibody response against it and the monoclonal antibody would then lose its value, having been neutralized by the antibody produced against it. To avoid this problem, researchers have developed techniques to replace all but those parts of the mouse antibody essential for its binding activity with sequences from human antibodies in a technique called *humanizing*. Sometimes, it is possible to develop fully human monoclonal antibodies by immunizing mice that have been genetically manipulated so that their genes for mouse antibodies have been replaced by genes for human antibodies. Other techniques for making human monoclonal antibodies also exist.

Monoclonal antibodies have been found to be extremely valuable as therapeutics. The Food and Drug Administration has approved at least thirty different monoclonal antibodies for the treatment of autoimmune diseases, cancer, heart disease, macular degeneration, transplant rejection, and other conditions. Indeed, monoclonal antibodies are among the "hottest" areas for drug development.

For example, the monoclonal antibody Herceptin (trade name for trastuzumab), specific for the oncoprotein Her2/neu, found on a subset of breast cancers usually associated with a poor prognosis, has been proven to be of substantial value in treating patients with recurrent cancers that express Her2/neu; it also has been shown valuable for initial treatment, in association with surgery and chemotherapy. In 2011, the monoclonal antibody ipilimumab specific for the T-cell surface protein CTLA-4 was approved for treatment of metastatic melanoma, where it has had a more impressive effect than any other single therapy, and it is being actively tested in a series of other cancers.

The potential for future application of monoclonal antibodies can hardly be overestimated. Many monoclonals are now in the drug development pipelines of pharmaceutical and biotech firms and surely more will enter these pipelines in the coming years.

Specific Types of Infections, Specific Types of T-Cell Responses

Infectious agents have evolved that can find a "home" in virtually every environment in the human body. These agents are disease-causing (pathogenic) for very different reasons. For example, many viruses are directly toxic to the cells they infect, causing tissue damage because they destroy cells. Some bacteria grow in the extracellular fluid and need to be controlled because their products or the response to them will compromise organ function. Other bacteria enter cells and live within them, often altering their function or leading to their death. Parasitic worms can establish infections in the gastrointestinal tract, the lung, or the liver and cause injury by evoking tissue-damaging inflammatory responses. Each of these infectious agents requires a different type of immune response if the infection is to be controlled and the pathogen eliminated.

We have seen how the process of determining the class of antibody that is made represents one form of appropriateness. Let us now consider appropriateness in terms of T-cell responses.

Richard Locksley, a physician-scientist working in the Department of Medicine at the University of California, San Francisco, was intrigued that some strains of mice infected in the foot pad with protozoan parasite *Leishmania major* could control the infection while others could not. When Locksley inoculated mice with leishmania, their foot pads swelled as parasites expanded in number. Some mice were able to eliminate the microorganisms, heal, and return to their normal state ("healer" mice). In other mice, however, the expansion of the parasite continued unchecked, eventually leading to the animals' death ("progressor" mice). Locksley considered the possibility that progressors did not make an immune response to the parasite, but he was able to show that was not the case; mice of progressor inbred strains made a robust T-cell response. In a landmark 1989 paper,[1] Locksley demonstrated that what was different between the healer mice and the progressors was not their degree of immunity to the parasite but the type of that immunity.

The healer mice made a CD4 T-cell response dominated by cells that produced the cytokine IFNγ. IFNγ has many properties; one of the most important is that it acts on macrophages to increase their capacity to kill microorganisms they have "eaten." The ability to kill the leishmania is one of the properties of IFNγ-stimulated macrophages. By contrast, the CD4 T cells that had responded to leishmania in the progressor mice failed to make IFNγ; in its place they produced large amounts of interleukin-4. If progressor mice were treated with an antibody that neutralizes IL-4, they then produced IFNγ and became healers, providing strong evidence that it is the different pattern of cytokines produced by healer and progressor CD4 T cells that determines their status.

When naïve CD4 T cells are activated by recognizing their cognate peptide-MHC complex on an activated dendritic cell, they not only begin to divide rapidly but also undergo a series of changes. Among these is that they acquire the capacity to produce different sets of cytokines. Activated CD4 T cells that can make IFNγ are designated *Th1* (T helper type 1) cells while those that make IL-4 are designated *Th2* cells. Which particular set of cytokines the differentiating CD4 T cell will be able to make is determined both by the precise conditions of the priming event and by the genetic constitution of the responding individuals.

Clearly then the type of CD4 T-cell response that an animal makes when infected with *Leishmania major* determines whether that animal will live or die. Despite making a very robust response, progressor mice generally are unable to control the parasite because their T cells have not differentiated into cells that could control the infection, as the cells of infected healer mice had. Rather, the cells from the progressor mice developed an entirely different fate, a Th2 fate, one that is ineffective in controlling the parasite.

We now recognize that naïve CD4 T cells have the potential to differentiate not only into Th1 and Th2 cells, the former marked by the ability to make IFNγ while the latter is characterized by the ability to make IL-4 and a series of related cytokines, but that other differentiation fates also exist.

These include cells that make the cytokine IL-17, often referred to as Th17 cells, and cells that can make IL-22, called by some Th22 cells. Naïve CD4 T cells can also develop into Tregs, although these Tregs have some properties that distinguish them from the Tregs that develop in the thymus.

These different types of Th cells have different roles. Th1 cells, good producers of IFNγ, are critical to the development of immune responses against intracellular bacteria, such as the tubercle bacillus, and to many viruses, as well as to leishmania. Their effectiveness against these pathogens can be attributed to the ability of IFNγ both to enhance the capacity of macrophages to kill ingested bacteria and other microorganisms and to cause the cell to express molecules that limit the capacity of viruses to survive within them.

Th2 cells are important in protection against infections with parasitic worms known as helminths, a group that includes hookworms and schistosomes. Th17 cells are critical in immune responses against extracellular bacteria, such as staphylococci, and against fungi.

This description of the specialized T-cell responses to distinct infectious challenges by no means exhausts the diversity of an individual's options. For example, CD8 T cells can make a variety of additional responses to pathogens. What is central is the concept of appropriateness: the immune system tailors responses to optimally control the threat a particular pathogen poses.

18

Our Discovery of IL-4 and the Cells

That Make It

At about the same time that Mark Davis was at work cloning the TCRβ chain in the Laboratory of Immunology (chapter 12), I was working to understand how B lymphocytes became activated. We knew that B cells had cell surface antibody-like molecules, and we had shown that when these molecules were engaged by their cognate antigen, changes occurred in the cell indicating that the biochemical pathways leading to B-cell activation had been triggered. These results showed that the membrane immunoglobulin of the B cells was a true signal-transducing receptor, the B-cell receptor.

To activate the B cells in tissue culture, my colleagues and I stimulated them with an antibody that could bind to membrane-bound IgM, one of the major BCRs of naïve B cells (the other was membrane IgD). We found that taking B cells from the lymph nodes or spleens of normal mice and culturing them with anti-IgM antibody caused the cells to divide. We measured this by our favorite method, the uptake of radioactively labeled thymidine.

When Maureen Howard, a postdoctoral fellow from the Hall Institute who had done her PhD work under the supervision of Burnet's protégé Gus Nossal, joined my laboratory, we decided to study B-cell activation in greater detail. We were immediately confronted with a problem, however. To study the response of lymphocytes in tissue culture, we placed the cells into culture wells, added anti-IgM antibody, and measured the results two or three days later by determining how much radioactive thymidine had been taken up by the cells in the culture well. What we found was the amount of radioactive thymidine taken up *per cell* diminished as the number of cells placed in an individual well diminished.

Of course, we had anticipated that as we reduced the number of cells in the tissue culture well, stimulation with anti-IgM would result in less radioactive thymidine uptake, but we expected that if we divided that amount of radioactive thymidine uptake by the number of cells in the well, the quotient would change very little as we changed the cell number. That is, we anticipated that the amount of thymidine taken up per cell would be independent of the number of cells cultured. What we observed, however, was that the quotient fell dramatically as we reduced the number of cells in the culture well.

This could be explained if the response of the B cells to anti-IgM antibody depended on or was helped by the product of another cell present in the culture well. If two cells are required to mediate a response, reducing the total number of cells twofold should not halve the response but should reduce the response by a factor of four as the likelihood of the cells interacting would be related to the frequency of each cell. Because halving a cell number reduces the frequency of each interacting cell twofold, the likelihood of an interaction occurring, which should be the product of the frequencies of the two cells, is reduced fourfold. That realization led us to consider the possibility that a second cell, probably a T cell in the culture, was important in the response of B cells to anti-IgM antibodies. One possible mechanism through which the T cells could work in this manner was by making a factor that would enhance the B cell's response.

To test this hypothesis, we placed B cells in culture at low cell density and then added culture fluid from a T-cell line in order to see whether the added culture fluid increased the uptake of radioactive thymidine when we stimulated the cells with anti-IgM. To our pleasure, we found that culture fluid from the mouse T-cell tumor line EL-4 caused a striking increase in the response of the B cells to anti-IgM antibody, implying that there was a factor made by EL-4 cells (and presumably normal T cells) that helped B cells respond.

Maureen and I, with a new postdoc, Junichi Ohara, used a variety of techniques to purify the substance in this EL-4 culture fluid and were able to show that it was a factor that had a molecular weight of 18,000 daltons. Junichi brought the factor to chemical purity and determined its sequence of amino acids. This molecule became known as interleukin-4. IL-4 is a member of a cytokine family that has a common overall structure and whose receptors are also similar in structure. They are often referred as type I cytokines.

The first function Maureen and I identified for IL-4 was that of helping B cells grow in response to anti-IgM. In collaborative experiments with Ellen Vitetta at the University of Texas Southwestern Medical Center in Dallas and with Bob Coffman in Palo Alto, we showed that IL-4 also mediates the immunoglobulin class switching of B cells from the expression of IgM to IgG1 and IgE (see chapter 16). Furthermore, IL-4 acts on other cell types to mediate many of the effects associated with allergies and asthma, as well as to provide a protective immune response to infection with parasitic worms, such as hookworm.

After we had identified and purified IL-4, Tim Mosmann and Bob Coffman, working at the DNAX Research Institute, now part of Merck, showed that different Th cells could be distinguished because they made different sets of cytokines. It was Mosmann and Coffman who first recognized that such distinctive sets of differentiated T cells (such as Th1, Th2, Th17, Th22, and induced Tregs) existed. They had prepared a series of T-cell lines that they carried in tissue culture over long periods of time. These cells could be activated by one of several different techniques. They found that they could classify most of their cell lines by virtue of the pattern of cytokines they produced. One set were good producers of IFNγ. They designated these Th1 cells. The other set of lines produced IL-4 and were designated Th2 cells. More than a decade would pass before other scientists established the existence of Th17 and Th22 cells.

After Mosmann and Coffman showed that primed CD4 T cells existed in at least two different states, the ball returned to our court. We asked, what determines the type of Th cell a naïve CD4 T cell will become when it responds to antigen? Graham LeGros, a postdoctoral fellow from New Zealand, and Zami Ben-Sasson, an Israeli scientist who had been a postdoc years earlier and continued to work closely with me while also being a Professor at the Hebrew University Hadassah Medical Center, jointly solved this problem. They made the striking finding that stimulating naïve CD4 T cells with an antibody to the TCR would cause those cells to differentiate into Th2 cells only if we included IL-4 in the culture medium. That is, the major product of the Th2 cells, IL-4, was also a major determinant of the type of Th cell a naïve CD4 T cell would become when it was primed. There was a positive feedback loop that would strikingly bias cells that had begun to differentiate in the Th2 direction to complete that differentiation. Thereafter, we and others showed that the principle of positive feedback in Th differentiation was general. Thus, Th1 cell differentiation depended on IFNγ, the cytokine that was the principal product of Th1 cells. A similar process works for Th17 cells, although it is somewhat indirect.   .

Thus, a line of work that began with our lab's effort to understand the mechanism controlling B cell responses to anti-IgM antibodies ended with a general principle underlying the differentiation of naïve CD4 T cells to various types of Th cells.

19

CD8 T Cells

Killer Cells and Friends

I have already discussed the distinct functions of different classes of antibodies and the mechanisms through which the nature of the immune response determines which class of antibody the immune system produces (or, more accurately, how a determination is made of to which class the B cell switches). We also know that switching occurs in a specialized location, the germinal centers of the lymph nodes and spleen. Switching depends on the properties of the particular Tfh cells that migrate into the germinal center and are thus present to "help" the B cell undergo the class switch process.

So when a CD4 T cell is primed by antigen, the conditions of this priming determine the "fate" of the responding CD4 T cells, inducing the different types of Th cells (e.g., Th1, Th2, Th17, Th22, Tfh). The choice of the fate of the responding CD4 T cell is important to the response because cells that adopt different characteristics are effective against certain classes of infections but may be essentially useless against other types of infection. A Th2-dominated response protects mice against infection with helminthic parasites but if mounted in leishmania infections allows the numbers of parasites to keep increasing, with the outcome being the death of the infected mouse. Thus, the determination of what type of cell a naïve CD4 T cell will become when it is primed by antigen is an example of appropriateness.

CD8 T cells act to protect us against infection and tumors using a range of responses. Recall that T cells that express receptors consisting of α and β chains come in two distinct forms, CD4 T cells and CD8 T cells. As we have seen, CD4 T cells recognize peptide-MHC complexes in which the

MHC molecule was of the class II type whereas CD8 T cells recognize peptide–class I MHC complexes.

This distinctive pattern of recognition has important implications because class I MHC molecules are widely expressed, even on cells of the central nervous system, whereas class II MHC molecules have a much more limited pattern of expression, being confined mainly to cells of the immune system. This is consistent with the function of the CD4 T cells, which work mainly by interacting with other cells of the immune system. This interaction is the means through which the CD4 T cells help B cells to develop into antibody-producing cells, assist macrophages to more efficiently destroy microbes that they have eaten, and aid dendritic cells to become better antigen-presenting cells. Thus, the CD4 T cell's function is to a large degree mediated by its recognition of peptide-MHC complexes on the surface of other cells of the immune and inflammatory systems, cells with which the CD4 T cell will "collaborate."

Because class I MHC molecules are expressed on the great majority of cells, not just the cells of the immune system, CD8 T cells have a much wider range of cells that they can "see" (by which I mean on which they identify their peptide-MHC complexes). In principle, the CD8 T cell's TCR can recognize its cognate antigen (i.e., peptide-MHC complex) on virtually any cell in the body that expresses the proper peptide product derived from a virus, bacteria, tumor antigen, or indeed any antigen that gains access to the cytoplasm of the cell. But what is the outcome of such recognition?

Another important difference between the CD4 and CD8 T cells is their functions. While CD8 T cells can produce cytokines, particularly IFNγ, just as CD4 T cells do, many of them also can kill cells that express a peptide-MHC complex that their TCRs can recognize.

Let's go into this killing function in a little more detail. First, naïve CD8 T cells generally lack killer activity. They need to be stimulated by encounter with their cognate antigen (a peptide–class I MHC complex) on the surface of an antigen-presenting dendritic cell. Once stimulated, the majority of the CD8 T cells develop into what are termed *effector* cells. Depending on the conditions of priming, these effectors may acquire the capacity to kill any cell that expresses the peptide-MHC complex that their TCRs can recognize.

The first step in this killing process is antigen-recognition. Because CD8 T cells attack only those cells that express peptides derived from the infecting pathogen that originally led to their priming, "off-target" or by-stander killing is strictly limited. As a result of the recognition step, bio-chemical events occur within the CD8 T cells that cause them first to express and then to secrete a molecule, *perforin*, that pokes holes in the membrane of the cells to which the killer cell has bound. Once it was thought that these holes were enough to kill the target cell, but now we recognize that the hole-punching is only part of the process. It is followed by the injection into the target cell of a potent enzyme, granzyme B, which cleaves proteins in the target cell, most importantly a set of molecules called *pro-caspases*. The cleaving of key pro-caspases produces enzymes (caspases) whose action signals the target cells to undergo apoptosis, or programmed cell death. Basically, the target cell commits suicide under instruction from the killer cell.

What is the value of such killing? Destroying a tumor cell is obviously advantageous. Moreover, it is evolutionarily useful for cells of the body to be prepared to undergo programmed cell death on "instruction" from a killer cell that has discovered that the target cell expresses a tumor antigen and thus is likely to be cancerous.

A similar situation exists for virus-infected cells. When viruses enter cells, their genetic material often takes over the protein-producing apparatus of the infected cell to produce more viruses of the same type, which would thus infect more cells, leading to greater and greater degrees of infection. If the killer cell can detect and destroy the virus-infected cell before it has produced new viruses, it can interrupt the infection.

How does this work? The goal of the killer cell is to recognize peptides produced in response to instructions from the virus *before* any intact new viruses are made. If the killer cell is successful in this identification, it can kill virus-infected cells before they have an opportunity to produce new viruses and infect additional cells.

There is, however, a potential danger in this strategy of killing virus-infected cells. If the killer cells fall behind the production of infectious virus, many cells can become infected before the killers are effective. Under such circumstances, the killer cells might destroy a large number of cells of a particular type. If these cells have an important function, then the immune response may lead to the loss of that function by killing so many of the infected cells. This process is referred to as *immunopathology*. If these cells have been infected with a virus that would destroy them (such viruses are often called *lytic viruses*), one could argue that the immunopathologic damage is a price worth paying. But not all viruses kill the cells they have infected. Some viruses lead to chronic infections in which the infected cell is still functional although probably not fully normal. In this instance, if the killer response is delayed, then the immune system can destroy an entire organ that would have continued to function, even if infected.

An example of immunopathologic damage caused by an exuberant CD8 T-cell response is chronic hepatitis B infection. In this disease, the virus itself does not destroy liver cells, the immune response does. The immunopathologic response may lead to cirrhosis of the liver and the attendant inflammation may contribute to the development of liver cancer in individuals with chronic hepatitis B infection.

A challenge for the immune system is to destroy cells infected with lytic viruses before they have infected too large a proportion of the cells of a given type while restraining overexuberant responses against nonlytic viruses and thus avoiding the immunopathology that would have occurred.

The immune system has evolved a mechanism to help to limit the immunopathology caused by a very strong CD8 T-cell response against nonlytic viruses. This mechanism can be illustrated by considering the outcome of infecting adult mice with the lymphocytic choriomeningitis virus (LCMV). There are two closely related forms of LCMV, Armstrong[1] and Clone 13. Mice infected with the Armstrong strain of LCMV make an immune response that rapidly eliminates the virus, but mice of the same inbred strain infected with the Clone 13 virus mount an immune response that is less effective and allows the virus to persist for a long period. Such viral persistence is precisely the circumstance in which a continued robust killer T-cell response or continued production of inflammatory cytokines such as IFNγ could cause severe immunopathology. In Clone 13 infection, the responding T cells are rendered unable to mediate effector functions, both killer function and IFNγ production, presumably to avoid the severe immunopathology that would occur if they remained active killer cells or IFNγ producers. The blockade of killer or IFNγ-producing activity among the responding CD8 cells in the Clone 13–infected mice is due to the expression on their surface of a molecule known as PD-1. PD-L1, a protein that binds to PD-1 and transmits signals through PD-1, is heavily expressed on macrophages, suggesting that the interaction of macrophages with

PD-1-expressing CD8 cells leads to their inactivation, thus avoiding the immunopathology that the activated cells might have caused.

The immune system obviously is making some difficult decisions. Whether it has a mechanism to distinguish infections with viruses that themselves cause cell death and those that do not is not yet clear. Avoiding unnecessary immunopathology by restraining a response against a non-lytic virus makes sense but "giving up" the effort to control a virus that itself destroys infected cells would be a serious blunder.

The discovery that interactions between PD-L1 and PD-1 restrain effector CD8 T cells in chronic viral infections suggested that blocking PD-1 might allow robust effector responses against antigens that for one reason or another have been suppressed by the PD-1 system. This appears to be the case particularly with immune responses to tumors. Some tumors of humans, including lung, ovarian, and colon, as well as melanomas, have been shown to express large amounts of PD-L1, consistent with their having the capacity to restrain cytotoxic responses that might have killed the tumor cells. Recent trials in humans with various cancers have shown that monoclonal antibodies that block PD-1 (lambrolizumab and nivolumab) and thus block the inactivation of CD8 T cells are highly effective anti-tumor agents. They allow the immune response to proceed against tumors that had restrained such responses by stimulation of PD-1. More precisely, these antibodies, by blocking the PD-1/PD-L1 interactions, allow T cells that had been primed by the tumor cells and then inactivated by PD-1/PD-L1 interaction to regain their responsiveness and to destroy the tumor cells. This type of immunologic manipulation, also shown by the monoclonal antibody to the cell surface protein CTLA-4 (ipilimumab), has been termed *checkpoint* therapy and promises to revolutionize treatment of certain cancers.

20

Dendritic Cells

The Cells That Interpret the Infectious Threat

It is important for T cells to distinguish between dangerous and innocuous antigens and then to make a response or not, as would be appropriate. When the decision is to make a response, the nature of that response (i.e., whether it is appropriate to the threat) is equally important. The survival or death of mice infected with leishmania depended on whether the responding T cells produced IFNγ or IL-4.

What determines whether a T cell will be activated and, if it is, how it will differentiate? A large element in this process is the action of the specialized population of cells, the dendritic cells.

Dendritic cells are stellate-shaped cells found in virtually every tissue in the body. The process of infection, either directly or indirectly, activates these cells. How they become activated will account for much of their fate. In chapter 15, when I presented my view of the mechanism of action of Tregs, I discussed the suppression of dendritic cell function by these regulatory cells. Dendritic cells are clearly central players in many aspects of T-cell activation.

Dendritic cells were discovered in 1973 by Ralph Steinman, working in the laboratory headed by Zanvil Cohn at the Rockefeller University. Steinman was a Canadian who had come to Cohn's laboratory after having been trained at Harvard Medical School and the Massachusetts General Hospital. Cohn's laboratory was perhaps the leading one in the world in which to study the properties of macrophages, and a large proportion of the leaders in the field of macrophage biology are graduates of this laboratory. In the course of Steinman's work, he noticed in the spleen and lymph

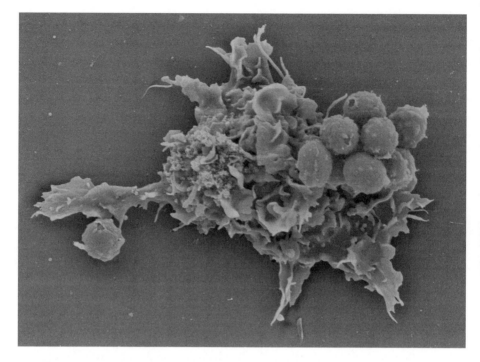

Figure 20.1. A dendritic cell with adherent lymphocytes. (Courtesy of Professor Matthias Gunzer, University of Duisburg-Essen, Germany)

nodes the presence of a highly stellate cell (figure 20.1) that had not previously been described, or at least to which no one had given proper attention.

To assess the function of these cells, Steinman had to purify them. Here he was very fortunate in his location because the Rockefeller University was the home of the research group that had originated the modern study of the various components (the organelles) of the cell. That group, headed by the Nobel laureate George Palade, had developed powerful methods to separate organelles. Steinman was able to adapt these techniques to purifying the relatively rare dendritic cells in lymph nodes and spleen from the much more numerous lymphocytes and macrophages.

Once Steinman had dendritic cells in enriched form, he could test them for various functions. Over several years of persistent effort, often in the face of a lack of encouragement from other immunologists, he showed that dendritic cells were the most potent antigen-presenting cells. Until Steinman's work, most immunologists believed that the macrophage was the principal cell for the presentation of the peptide-MHC complex to the T cell. This view was based on the observation that cells from the spleen and lymph node that could adhere to tissue culture wells had excellent antigen-presenting ability. The great majority of these cells were macrophages.

But these adherent cells were far from pure populations. Among the cells that also adhered to tissue culture dishes were dendritic cells. Steinman compared purified macrophages and dendritic cells to each other in their capacity to activate T cells, as measured by antigen-stimulated uptake of radioactive thymidine. The dendritic cells proved to be fifty times more potent, on a per cell basis, than the macrophages.

This observation attracted the attention of many scientists, and the dendritic cell became a "star" and has been studied extremely intensively. It was quickly shown that dendritic cells were not a homogeneous population. Rather, they consisted of several different cell types with distinctive functions and distinctive locations. It was further shown that the dendritic cell was the bridge between innate immune responses, triggered by the sensing of pathogens or of danger signals, and the activation of the key cells of the adaptive immune system, the CD4 T cells.

For example, infection with certain viruses or challenging an animal with an analog of viral RNA, polyinosinic:polycytydilc acid (polyI:C), often elicits a dendritic cell response in which type I interferons[1] and the cytokine interleukin-12 (IL-12) are made, mainly by dendritic cells. Dendritic cells of this type are very good at activating naïve CD4 T cells to become Th1 cells, which make large amounts of IFNγ. IFNγ acts to enhance the capacity of cells to prevent viral replication and thus such a response can be quite effective in controlling infections with viruses such as influenza. Other methods of activating dendritic cells can yield cells that are much more effective in causing naïve CD4 T cells to differentiate to Th17 or Th2 cells. Thus, how the dendritic cell is activated (or possibly, which of several different types of dendritic cells are activated) profoundly alters the fate chosen by T cells responding to the antigen presented by those dendritic cells and will influence the protective value of those T cells.

In an effort to improve vaccine effectiveness, several groups have taken advantage of the function of dendritic cells as potent antigen-presenting cells. Rather than simply injecting the vaccine in a soluble form or perhaps in association with an approved adjuvant such as alum, researchers have allowed antigen to be taken up by dendritic cells in tissue culture and have then injected those "antigen-loaded" dendritic cells into animals in an effort to enhance the immunogenicity of weak vaccines. While this technology has not yet reached the stage that it could be thought of for routine use in humans, it has been used in many experimental settings. In general, antigen-loaded dendritic cells have been an effective way to increase the efficacy of weak vaccines.

Ironically, Ralph Steinman developed pancreatic cancer in 2003. After surgery, he worked with colleagues in an attempt to induce an immune response to his cancer by preparing dendritic cells from his blood and then loading them with tumor lysates in the hope that injecting them would induce a robust immunity against residual cancer cells. Whether the vaccine attempts worked or not was never clear, but Steinman survived with his cancer for eight years, far longer than the average patient with pancreatic malignancy.

Indeed, it wasn't until September 30, 2011, on a Friday, that Ralph lost his battle with his disease. On the following Monday, October 3, the Nobel Prize in Physiology or Medicine for 2011 was announced, and Ralph was one of the laureates. The Nobel committee had not been aware of his death just three days earlier, and after a brief uncertainty, the decision was that the award would stand, although the rules generally state that Nobel Prizes cannot be posthumous. But the committee must have concluded the decision to award him a share of the prize was made while he was alive, and it was only the announcement that occurred after his death. Thus, one of the truly innovative discoveries of modern immunology received its well-deserved recognition, although Steinman's discovery of dendritic cells would stand as a great accomplishment with or without the recognition by the Nobel committee.

V HOW DID THE IMMUNE SYSTEM EVOLVE?

An "Ancient" Immune Response Controls "Modern" Immunity

Dendritic cells interpret the nature of the microbial or danger threat and then make a response. That response determines the type of effector function adopted by antigen-specific CD4 T cells when they are stimulated by peptide-MHC complexes presented by those dendritic cells. But what is it that the dendritic cells recognize that allows them to determine the nature of the microbial threat? What is the consequence of such "threat recognition"?

PAMPs and PRRs

This story starts with a proposal in 1989 by Charles Janeway. Janeway was a leading immunologist and a professor at Yale. Years earlier, he had come to the National Institutes of Health as a postdoctoral fellow in my research group. Charlie worked with me for five years. He was clearly an individual of great creativity, but his five years in Bethesda, although well spent and productive, did not give a hint as to how he would later upset the immunological apple cart.

Charlie came from a distinguished medical family. His great-grandfather, Edward Gamaliel Janeway, was the health commissioner of New York City from 1875 to 1882 and was Professor of Pathology and Practical Anatomy at Bellevue Hospital Medical College, one of the antecedents of the New York University School of Medicine. Charlie's grandfather, Theodore Caldwell Janeway, was the first full-time professor of medicine at the Johns Hopkins School of Medicine. The Janeway lesion, a sign of bacterial endocarditis, is named for him. Charlie's father, Charles Alderson Janeway, was an eminent pediatrician who was physician-in-chief at Children's

Hospital of Boston from 1946 to 1976 and is regarded as one of the founders of the study of immunodeficiency diseases.

Charlie joined my group in July 1970 after graduating from Harvard Medical School and completing an internship at the Peter Bent Brigham Hospital (now Brigham and Women's Hospital). He had taken time during medical school to do research in the United Kingdom with two of the leading British immunologists, John Humphrey and Robin Coombs, and had come to NIH fully expecting to work under the supervision of Baruj Benacerraf. But, as I recounted earlier, Baruj left for Harvard on June 30, 1970, one day before Charlie's arrival.

Shortly after getting started in my lab, Charlie received a formal letter from Dorland Davis, the director of the National Institute of Allergy and Infectious Diseases, asking him to serve on the institute's council, which was its most senior advisory body. It quickly became clear that the letter was meant for his father and had come to Charlie through a clerical error. Nonetheless, it resulted in my having the opportunity to meet with the elder Janeway, whose principal concern was that I "look after his boy." Needless to say, Charlie was quite able to take that responsibility on his own, but we spent five delightful and exciting years together.

The great questions of the first century of immunology were how specificity was achieved (comprising the study of the first law, universality) and how responses against our own tissues were avoided (the second law, tolerance). Not a lot of attention had been given to the problem of how the immune response was regulated so that it would be appropriate to the threat (appropriateness). How was it that a viral infection would elicit an immune response dominated by Th1 cells, the production of IFNγ, and of cytotoxic T cells while an infection with extracellular bacteria, such as pneumococci, would lead to a response dominated by Th17 cells and by the production of antibodies capable of promoting macrophage phagocytosis of organisms coated with those antibodies?

In my presidential address to the American Association of Immunologists in 1987, I grappled with exactly this issue.[1] I argued that the period from the Pasteur discovery that infection with attenuated bacteria protected against infection with a virulent bacterium of the same type to the date of the lecture, the overwhelming body of work in immunology had been devoted to the problem of specificity and its logical partner, tolerance.

I further argued that the pendulum was swinging very strongly to the study of how the immune response was regulated, how responses that were appropriate to the threat were controlled.

Charlie took up this challenge and confronted what has often been called the immunologist's "dirty little secret," the secret being that foreign substances injected into an individual did not give a robust immune response unless an "adjuvant" was also administered. At the time, little was understood about what adjuvants did. In humans, many vaccines were given with the only FDA-approved adjuvant at the time, alum, a sulfate salt of potassium and aluminum. Alum existed in a crystalline form, which would later be thought to be important for its adjuvant activity. But at the time, it was simply known that adsorbing antigen onto alum would strikingly increase the immune response against the antigen.

In a famous lecture delivered at an influential 1989 meeting held at the Cold Spring Harbor Laboratory, on Long Island, New York, Charlie made a proposal that would provide the underpinning for all subsequent work in the field.[2] In many respects, his proposal was quite simple, but it nicely fits a quote from Albert Szent-Györgyi: "Discovery consists of seeing what everyone else has seen and thinking what nobody else has thought."[3]

Charlie argued that the immune system makes a decision whether it should respond to a foreign antigen, an antigen for which both T cells and B cells exist that have receptors that can bind to antigenic determinants of or derived from the antigen. That decision is based on the innate immune system's recognition of specific microbial products that are so central to the survival of the microorganism that it could not exist without them and thus could not escape stimulating the immune system. Charlie called such substances pathogen-associated molecular patterns (PAMPs), and he designated the receptors that recognized the PAMPs *pattern recognition receptors* (PRRs). The basic notion was that a PAMP interacting with a PRR would stimulate an adjuvant-like activity and would allow a foreign antigen to elicit a robust immune response. Thus, a recognition event mediated by a PAMP interacting with a PRR would condition the interaction of specific T cells with their cognate peptide-MHC complexes presented by dendritic cells to lead to a robust T-cell response. The same could be said for B cells responding to the three-dimensional structure for which they were specific (see chapter 16).

Interleukin-1 and Drosophila Toll

To discuss how we moved from the PAMP-PRR proposal to an actual understanding of the adjuvant process, let's look at a particular adjuvant, bacterial lipopolysaccharide (LPS). LPS is a component of the outer membrane of a class of microorganisms called *gram-negative bacteria*.[4] LPS is a complex of a large polysaccharide and fatty acids, which are acids with long lipid "tails." LPS coadministered with antigens strikingly enhances the immune response to those antigens. It was believed that the PAMP-PRR problem might be easier to "crack" through the study of LPS than the study of the other popular adjuvants because there were two inbred strains of mice that were unresponsive to LPS but could respond to other adjuvants. Their specific unresponsiveness to LPS had been shown by breeding experiments to be the consequence of a mutation in a single gene. If the gene could be identified, then there was a good chance that one could determine how the product of that gene, which might be a PRR, caused a greater immune response when engaged by the PAMP, in this case LPS. Indeed, this proved to be the case, but the story of how we got to that understanding, as always, is convoluted.

It begins with the study of the cytokine interleukin-1 (IL-1), which causes a variety of inflammatory responses; it is one of a group of pro-inflammatory cytokines. Now, the term *interleukin* means a protein that acts *between* leukocytes (white blood cells). This is a very general term used for a wide variety of proteins made by leukocytes that act on other leukocytes and, in many cases, on other types of cells. There are currently thirty-six molecules with interleukin designations (IL-1 to IL-36).[5] IL-1 was one of the earliest to be discovered, and it was given the "1" designation because of what appeared to be an important function in T-cell development that occurred earlier in the development process than did a function mediated by a second molecule being studied at the same time, which accordingly received the name IL-2. (IL-2, remember, is important for the survival and function of Tregs.)

IL-1 is made by many cell types and has many functions. Indeed, my colleagues and I have shown that it can act as an exceedingly potent adjuvant,[6] but this aspect of its function was not generally emphasized in the late 1980s.

Those studying how IL-1 mediated its function had uncovered important details of the signaling pathway through which IL-1 had its impact on its target cells. First, it was known that IL-1 bound to a cell surface receptor called IL-1 receptor 1 (IL-1R1). IL-1R1 extends into the cytoplasm of the target cell, and that extension has an important structural characteristic, a stretch of amino acids now called a *TIR domain*. (More on TIR domains below.) Another protein, Myd88, also containing a TIR domain, becomes bound to the IL-1R1 TIR domain when the cell is treated with IL-1. A consequence of IL-1 activating its target cells and bringing Myd88 in apposition to the IL-1R1 TIR domain was the recruitment of NF-κB, a transcription factor system that controls many inflammatory responses. Finally, an important effect of activating NF-κB in response to IL-1 was the production of several pro-inflammatory cytokines, particularly TNFα. Grasping this process is critical to solving the adjuvant puzzle.

The story now turns to the immune system of the fruit fly, *Drosophila melanogaster*. *Drosophila* has an immune system, but it lacks the modern components that include T cells, B cells, and antibodies. These components, of course, make up the adaptive immune system. The fly (and all invertebrates) has only an innate immune system.

Drosophila has been an extremely valuable organism for geneticists to use to study gene function. One of its genes was identified based on the fact that when it was mutated so that it could not function, the fly showed a failure to develop the normal up/down (dorsal/ventral) polarization of its body. It was designated the *toll* gene (German for great, amazing, or stunning).

Bruno Lemaitre and Jules Hoffmann, working in Strasbourg, had undertaken an effort to identify genes that were important in the capacity of *Drosophila* to resist certain infections. They were struck by the fact that toll, known for its effects on the development of the body plan of the fly, shared many properties with the mammalian IL-1 receptor.

The toll pathway consisted of a series of genes many of which had been identified. *Drosophila* geneticists establish a *pathway* when mutation of different genes leads to a very similar effect (a similar *phenotype*). Also, these geneticists often use picturesque names for their genes, sometimes descriptive of what a fly looks like or how it behaves when the gene is mutated.

Toll itself resembles IL-1R1 in that in its intracellular portion it has the amino acid signature of a TIR domain. Indeed, TIR stands for toll IL-1 receptor. When toll is activated by binding an extracellular molecule called *spätzle*, the TIR domain in its intracellular portion binds to the TIR domain of the molecule *pelle*. This resembles the interaction of the TIR domains of the intracellular portion of IL-1R1 and of Myd88. Finally, the recruitment of pelle to toll results in biochemical changes in the genes *cactus* and *dorsal*, which are homologs of two key protein components of the vertebrate NF-κB system, known to be activated by IL-1. The final step in the activation of the toll pathway in *Drosophila* is the production of the antifungal peptide drosomycin. Mutations in toll (or in other key members of the pathway) make the fly extremely susceptible to fungal infection.

Thus, through elegant genetic analysis of *Drosophila* genes, Lemaitre, Hoffmann, and their colleagues established that toll was a key player in the fly's innate immune system and, quite remarkably, that its mode of action had a very substantial resemblance to that of IL-1, a key pro-inflammatory cytokine of humans.

Toll-like Receptors

This work obviously demanded an effort to see whether toll existed in humans and other higher vertebrates. If it did, then what did it do? Janeway and Hoffmann had already recognized that a search in *Drosophila* for the molecules that mediated the fly's immune system could be very valuable. Janeway had been meeting regularly with Hoffmann and several other scientists to discuss how to tackle this problem.

After Lemaitre's paper appeared in the journal *Cell*,[7] Ruslan Medzhitov, a postdoctoral fellow in Charlie Janeway's research group at Yale, immediately began the search for human toll. He took advantage of a remarkable resource of the US National Library of Medicine. When new genes and their mRNA products are discovered and the sequence of nucleotides in them determined, that information is deposited in a database maintained by the library. Medzhitov immediately searched this database using powerful mathematical tools to ask whether there were any human genes that resembled *Drosophila* toll, particularly in its intracellular portion. Indeed, one homolog had been previously described; Medzhitov discovered a second with substantial homology.

He and Janeway were able to study the function of this human homolog of toll by introducing an engineered form of the gene into human cells and showing that when the resultant protein was activated, it caused the NF-κB system to be engaged and led to the production of key cytokines, precisely the behavior one might anticipate for molecules functioning as PRRs. Medzhitov and Janeway named this molecule human toll, but subsequently toll-like receptor (TLR) has been adopted to refer to this and a related set of molecules.

Medzhitov and Janeway's experiment demonstrated that the TLR(s) that existed in humans had properties that might be expected of a PRR, but it did not tell us whether it truly was a PRR since there was no information about what it recognized or whether it actually functioned physiologically as an adjuvant receptor. Furthermore, no clue would come from *Drosophila*. In contrast to the concept that PRRs recognize microbial products, toll recognized a protein of the fly itself, spätzle, not an exogenous microbial product. In that respect, toll was actually closer to the IL-1 receptor than to a PRR because the IL-1 receptor (the homolog of toll) recognizes an internal mammalian protein, IL-1. Thus, some new approach was needed to determine what the molecule was that the TLR recognized.

This brings us back to LPS and the two strains of mice genetically unable to respond to LPS. The test used to determine their unresponsiveness was the failure of LPS to induce production of the pro-inflammatory cytokine TNFα by macrophages.[8]

Bruce Beutler, a co-discoverer of TNFα, now at the University of Texas Southwestern Medical Center in Dallas, had set out to identify the gene that was defective in the mouse strains whose macrophages failed to produce TNFα when stimulated with LPS. He used a technique called *positional cloning* that, at that time, was tedious but very powerful. Basically, his positional cloning strategy involved breeding mice that are defective in the gene determining responsiveness to LPS (the defective form of the gene was designated LPS^d) to normal inbred mice (LPS^n), analyzing the second generation offspring (F2 mice) for the inheritance of two copies of the LPS^d gene (LPS$^{d/d}$) based on their inability to produce TNFα in response to LPS. By determining for a large number of LPS$^{d/d}$ mice, the allelic form of many marker genes they had co-inherited from the original LPS$^{d/d}$ strain, he identified a very small genetic region in which the LPS^d gene was located. Through a series of genetic strategies, Beutler found that LPS^d was, in fact, a defective form of the TLR that Medzhitov and Janeway had studied, by now designated TLR4, as other TLRs had been identified in the interval.

Thus, in this case, the PRR was TLR4, and the PAMP was LPS. Researchers quickly identified more TLRs. Humans have ten TLRs; mice have twelve. The PAMPs that each of these TLRs recognize also have been identified. They mainly represent microbial products so central to the survival of the microbe that they cannot be dispensed with. The TLRs provide a powerful system to sense distinct microbes (they are *microbial sensors*), and different TLRs sense different classes of microbes.

An example of how TLR recognition is not simply a determination of whether an adaptive response should or should not occur but rather what the nature of the response should be comes from the study of how TLR3 identifies its PAMP. TLR3 recognizes double-stranded RNA, RNA in which the two strands are complementary to one another and thus pair. Double-stranded RNA is the genetic material of a class of viruses that include reoviruses, which cause many respiratory infections, and rotavirus, a chief cause of infant diarrhea and a major killer in the developing world. TLR3 engagement leads to the production of type I interferons,[9] which in turn act on dendritic cells and cause them to produce IL-12. When T cells are primed in the presence of IL-12, they are biased to develop into Th1 cells, which produce IFNγ. The latter is important in controlling viral infections. Thus, TLR recognition plays an important role in determining that the response is appropriate to the threat.

Other Receptors

TLRs are not the only class of microbial sensors. In the explosion of research that has gone on since the discovery of human TLRs, several other molecular families of microbial sensors have been discovered. TLRs are positioned at the cell surface or, in some cases, in the vesicles that take up particles and proteins from the outside of the cell. Other microbial sensors exist within the cytoplasm of the infected cell and are specialized to detect microbes or the products of microbes that have gained access to the interior of cells. Among the most important of these are a family of molecules designated the *NOD-like receptors* (NLRs). NOD stands for nucleotide-binding oligomerization domain.

There are many NLRs, but one of the most important is NLRP3. Although precisely how NLRP3 recognizes various microbes and their products isn't completely clear, it is known that NLRP3 can be activated by viruses such as influenza and by bacteria that can gain access to the cytoplasm of the infected cell. Certain crystals can also activate the NLRP3 pathway. It has been suggested that this is how alum crystals act as adjuvants in the immune system, although this interpretation is still controversial. What is clear is that crystals formed from urates are potent activators of NLRP3. Urates and uric acid are the key agents that lead to gout. Gout is basically an inflammatory disorder in which urate crystals are deposited in the cells of joints and surrounding tissues and, as we now know, are recognized there by NLRP3. The consequence of this recognition is the activation of an inflammasome (see below) with the consequent production of IL-1β and other mediators of inflammation. Gout, therefore, is actually a disease of the overactivity of a PAMP-PRR system through urate crystals stimulation of NLRP3. Blocking the action of IL-1β with anakinra, a drug that prevents IL-1β from binding to IL-1R1, is a highly effective treatment for gout.

Cholesterol crystals can also activate NLRP3, leading to *inflammasome* activation and thus to local production of IL-1β and its attendant inflammation, particularly in blood vessel walls where it contributes to atherosclerosis. This is just one more example of the critical role the immune system plays in a wide range of diseases.

Inflammasomes

What is an inflammasome, and how does it work? The inflammasome is a multi-protein molecular complex that has the role of recognizing an intracellular PAMP and communicating that recognition to cause the production of IL-1β and other key pro-inflammatory mediators. NLRP3 is the component that gives it its name and, more importantly, determines the substances that activate the NLRP3 inflammasome. Activating NLRP3 recruits an adapter protein, ASC, which in turn recruits a potent enzyme, caspase 1, that can cleave other proteins. One protein that caspase 1 particularly targets is a precursor of IL-1β. IL-1β is made as a molecule termed pro-IL-1β, which has little or no biological activity but can be cleaved by caspase 1 to its active, mature form. A congener of IL-1β, IL-18, which is also pro-inflammatory although it generally acts on different cell types, is also produced as a result of caspase 1 cleaving its "pro-form" to produce the active cytokine.

Thus, activating NLRP3 with urate crystals leads to the assembly of the NLRP3 inflammasome, to the activation of caspase 1, to the cleavage of the inactive pro-forms of IL-1β and IL-18, with their consequent release and activation of a host of inflammatory products, and to the severe and exquisitely painful inflammation characteristic of gout.

Auto-inflammatory Diseases

Some patients suffer from auto-inflammatory diseases in which excess IL-1β is produced. One such auto-inflammatory disease is neonatal onset multisystem inflammatory disease (NOMID). NOMID is a rare disease that appears early in life. Affected children have skin lesions resembling hives, inflammatory arthritis, noninfectious meningitis, and a series of other abnormalities due to severe inflammation. In a majority of these children, the disease is caused by a mutation in NLRP3 that activates the NLRP3 inflammasome even if it is not engaged by one of its normal stimulants. The outcome is unrestrained production of IL-1β. Dan Kastner and his colleagues at NIH, who determined the genetic basis of NOMID and a series of related diseases, showed that treating these children with the drug anakinra, which works by preventing IL-1β from binding to IL-1R1, results in rapid and impressive improvement in virtually all aspects of the disease. If anakinra treatment is stopped the symptoms rapidly return.

The best known of the auto-inflammatory diseases is familial Mediterranean fever (FMF),[10] a disease common in certain Mediterranean populations, particularly among Sephardic Jews, in which there is periodic fever, severe abdominal pain, and joint inflammation. IL-1β production appears to be a major cause of FMF, and anakinra has been used to treat FMF.

Why Can't Microbes Avoid PRRs?

We all know that bacteria that once were highly susceptible to antibiotics have now become resistant. This occurs when a mutation in some critical gene in a rare bacteria occurs that makes that particular bacterium resistant to the antibiotic. Since all the other bacteria are killed or hampered in their growth by the antibiotic, the resistant ones take over. Thereafter, the antibiotic has very limited usefulness for treating infections caused by those resistant bacteria.

One would anticipate that bacteria and viruses that are detected by one of the inflammasomes would become resistant as a result of a comparable favorable mutation. Why hasn't this happened over the long millennia that humans and microbes have been living together? The current microbial sensors are specific for molecules that are essential for the pathogen's survival and cannot easily be changed by mutation and still retain their activity. Let's look at one case in detail to grasp why an infectious agent cannot avoid the "attention" of a microbial sensor.

One important PAMP recognized in the cytoplasm of cells is double-stranded DNA (dsDNA). That is DNA as it normally exists in our genome or in the genome of bacteria, and in an important class of viruses. A good example of dsDNA viruses is the family of herpes viruses, which include herpes simplex, the chicken pox virus, and choriomeningitis virus, which causes severe infections in patients with AIDS.

dsDNA from bacteria and viruses gains access to the cytoplasm where it may be recognized by an inflammasome, one in which the recognition element is AIM2 (the acronym is derived from "absent in melanoma 2"). The recognition of dsDNA by AIM2 (which gives its name to the inflammasome) is not determined by the sequence of the components (the nucleotides) of the dsDNA. The solution of the three-dimensional structure of AIM2 showed that it "reads" not the sequence of the nucleotides within the dsDNA but rather the series of electrical charges distributed over its surface that are intrinsic to DNA's basic structure. Thus, mutations that might allow a virus to avoid recognition would disrupt the fundamental structure of DNA and be incompatible with the survival of the virus.

Honeybees and Innate Immunity

We looked briefly at the innate immune system of insects as part of the story of the discovery of how pathogen-sensing regulates our immune system, but insect immunity has its own importance. A failure of innate immunity may be causing the worldwide decline in honeybee populations. Honeybees play a central role in many aspects of modern agriculture, carrying pollen (male haploid gametophytes) from the anther of one plant to the stigma of another. Honeybee pollination has immense importance for many crops of great commercial value. *Colony collapse disorder* over the last ten years or more has been responsible for the loss in some instances of 30 percent or more of hives in a single year. One explanation for this serious situation appears to be the decline of innate immunity in honeybees as a result of their exposure to sublethal amounts of the insecticide clothianidin, a member of the neonicotinoid family of insecticides.[11] The insecticide causes an increase in the expression of a protein designated DME/LRR. This protein inhibits the activation of NF-κB and thus diminishes the production of antimicrobial peptides such as drosomycin and defensins. The result of this is that deformed wing (DFW) viruses borne by the honeybee expand strikingly in affected insects. The resultant loss of honeybee hives indicates how important innate immunity is to the survival of insects in general and honeybees in particular.

Vitamin A Deficiency

Mobilizing an immune response has eradicated smallpox and rinderpest worldwide. Almost as impressive, however, as a public health intervention, is the use of vitamin A as a supplement for children growing up in the developing world.

This story starts with a young ophthalmologist, Alfred Sommer, who was interested in the problem of night blindness and xerophthalmia in the developing world. Xerophthalmia is a condition in which there is severe dryness of the cornea and conjunctiva. If untreated, it can progress to corneal ulceration and blindness. Xerophthalmia is due to severe vitamin A deficiency, and an early sign of vitamin A deficiency is night blindness.

In 1976, on finishing his residency in ophthalmology at the Wilmer Eye Institute of Johns Hopkins Medical School, Sommer went to Indonesia to study the prevalence of eye disease due to vitamin A deficiency. He found that xerophthalmia was widespread in the region where he worked, but the far more important story was the effect of more moderate vitamin A deficiency, which was very common in infants and children. Sommer observed that such moderate deficiency coincided with a markedly elevated death rate from infections, particularly measles. He suspected that the vitamin A deficiency was putting these children at risk of death to measles and to infection with microorganisms that cause diarrheal diseases.

To determine whether there was a cause and effect relationship between vitamin A deficiency and inability to deal with measles, Sommer organized a controlled trial in which he compared children who received vitamin A supplementation with children who had not. The results were striking; supplementation resulted in a marked diminution in measles fatalities, so marked that many considered that it would be unethical to conduct additional clinical trials elsewhere as the control group would be deprived of what is clearly a lifesaving intervention.

Thus, Sommer showed that this very inexpensive intervention markedly improved the ability of children in the developing world to survive a measles infection.[12] More recent analysis has indicated that vitamin A supplementation in *at risk* populations can reduce mortality among children from *all* causes by more than 20 percent.

The cost of delivery of vitamin A to a child for a year has been estimated at $1.20. The World Health Organization uses a statistic to measure the cost effectiveness of various interventions, the cost per *disability adjusted life year* (DALY) gained by the intervention. Vitamin A is one of the cheapest, if not the cheapest way to "buy" a DALY.

How does vitamin A contribute to resistance to measles? The effect involves both the adaptive and innate arms of the immune system. Vitamin A is metabolized in the body to retinoic acid. In turn, retinoic acid is recognized by a receptor that resembles the receptors for steroid hormones. The retinoic acid receptors are intracellular molecules that become transcription factors on binding of their target (retinoic acid).

Vitamin A / retinoic acid has many functions, regulating the migration of cells of the immune and inflammatory systems and the capacity of CD4 T cells to develop into effector cells, in particular to cells of the Th17 type. Much work still remains to understand how vitamin A action on the innate and T-cell system orchestrates the response that protects against measles and other infections. Nevertheless, despite our incomplete knowledge of the process, the great value of the intervention indicates the varied, and even unexpected, impact of the immune system on human health.

22

The Microbiome and Innate Immunity

Our intestines harbor an incredible number of different kinds of bacteria. Usually, we live with these organisms in a mutually beneficial relationship. For this reason, they are often described as *commensal*, a term one of whose meanings is "eating at the same table." Until recently, we did not appreciate how many different kinds of bacteria have taken up residence within us. The development of new techniques that allow the rapid sequencing of large numbers of different strands of RNA has given us a much truer picture of the diversity of these organisms. Many of them cannot be grown on the usual bacterial culture plates so that, until recently, we had no idea of their presence.

Microbiome Diversity

Keeping a normal distribution of intestinal bacteria, often called *microbiota*, is important. Treatment of infections with broad-spectrum antibiotics has the consequence that many of the bacteria in our intestines are eliminated. This sometimes allows a limited set of bacteria, sometimes only one type, to take over. A "bad" example that is all too common is the dominance of the intestinal microbiota by *Clostridium difficile* in antibiotic-treated patients, particularly in hospitalized individuals undergoing cancer chemotherapy who require aggressive treatment with broad-spectrum antibiotics. *C. dif*, as it is often referred to, can cause severe inflammation of the colon with production of toxins that can be life threatening. Treatment of *C. dif* is difficult and not always successful; it is a complication to be avoided if at all possible.

But the importance of the normal microbiota in the intestine goes well beyond the simple avoidance of *C. dif* infection. It is clear that some (perhaps, many) of the bacteria in our gut have extremely positive functions. When they are absent, the consequences can be severe. Similarly, it appears that we may harbor bacteria that can cause extremely serious abnormalities if left unchecked.

A good example of the differential effects of intestinal bacteria may be seen in certain experimental forms of inflammatory bowel disease. These diseases are laboratory models of human ulcerative colitis and Crohn's disease. As we have seen, naïve CD4 T cells can adopt different fates on activation, the chief examples being Th1, Th2, and Th17 cells. In this process the cells express transcription factors that regulate the pattern of gene expression in these distinct types. Such factors are referred to as "master regulators." For Th1 development, the master regulator is T-bet. Laurie Glimcher and her colleagues at the Harvard School of Public Health observed that mice that lacked T-bet, because of a genetically engineered disruption of the T-bet gene, were very susceptible to the development of colitis.

Although I pointed out that T-bet was critical in development of Th1 differentiation, it also functions in other cell types and regulates the capacity of those cells to function at the mucosal surface. Glimcher and her colleagues showed that the deficiency of T-bet in dendritic cells, not T cells, was the key to the development of this colitis. Without T-bet, the dendritic cells make excessive amounts of TNFα, which causes colonic inflammation.

But what is truly remarkable is that housing normal mice together with mice that are genetically defective in T-bet results in the normal mice developing the same type of colitis that occurs in the T-bet-deficient mice. We know that co-housed mice will acquire their microbiota from their cage partners. Thus, the susceptibility of the normal mice to colitis implies that the microbiota of the T-bet-deficient mice is important in inducing the colitis. The transfer of their microbiota to normal mice causes them to develop the same type of colitis even though they lack the genetic defect that predisposes to the colitis.

This is just one way the distinct functions of the microbiota affects overall health, influencing conditions we might not normally think were within the province of gut bacteria or of the innate immune system. This finding of the transfer of susceptibility to colitis from an animal with a genetic predisposition to developing colitis to an entirely normal animal illustrates that the abnormalities that give rise to the "pathogenic" microbiota need not be present for animals to develop the pathologic state as long as the "abnormal" gut bacteria are present.

The Innate Immune System, Fatty Liver, and Metabolic Syndrome

What does this all have to do with the immune system and with the microbial sensing? Experiments from the research group headed by Richard Flavell at the Yale University School of Medicine illuminate how such abnormalities develop and the role of innate immunity in this process. Flavell and his colleagues were interested in the development of an abnormality in which fat accumulates in the liver. In humans, nonalcoholic fatty liver is an increasingly common abnormality that predisposes to cirrhosis of the liver and also, although less frequently, to liver cancer. Nonalcoholic fatty liver is associated with *metabolic syndrome*, which consists of obesity, resistance to insulin, elevated blood lipids, and diabetes, or at least some of the early signs of predisposition to diabetes such as inability to control blood sugar levels (abnormal glucose tolerance). Metabolic syndrome and fatty liver are developing into very severe health problems in the western world.

Flavell and his colleagues observed that mice that are defective in the NLRP6 inflammasome are very susceptible to developing fatty liver in response to a diet that is used to induce this disorder. Mice deficient in the adapter protein ASC are, like NLRP6-deficient mice, highly susceptible to developing fatty liver. Activation of caspase 1, the terminal component of inflammasomes, leads to the production of mature IL-1β and its congener IL-18. Genetically engineered mice that are deficient in the receptor for IL-1β, and thus unresponsive to the cytokine, are not more susceptible to developing fatty liver than are normal mice, but IL-18-deficient mice are more susceptible. These observations imply that the production of IL-18 normally keeps in check some process that would make mice more susceptible to fatty liver and, as we will see, to the related metabolic syndrome.

What is IL-18 doing, and where does it do it? The abnormality in innate sensing in mice lacking NLRP6 or ASC that enhances susceptibility to fatty liver is not seen if the deletion of these genes is limited to either dendritic cells or liver cells. It seems likely that the defect in pathogen-sensing that makes the animal more susceptible to fatty liver is in cells of the intestinal tract. Mice that have defects in the NLRP6 inflammasome or in IL-18 production have an altered intestinal microbiota with more bacteria of certain types and fewer of other types.[1] Remarkably, just as Glimcher observed for susceptibility to colitis, housing mice with a genetically determined greater susceptibility to fatty liver disease together with normal mice led to the normal mice becoming more likely to develop fatty liver and metabolic syndrome. The normal mice acquire the altered intestinal microbiota seen in the genetically susceptible mice, suggesting that it is the microbiota that are ultimately critical to the development of fatty liver. Consistent with this conclusion is that treatment of the normal mice with broad spectrum antibiotics diminishes their acquired susceptibility to fatty liver.

So how does the altered microbiota lead to fatty liver? While this is still not fully understood, we do have pieces of the puzzle. The abnormal microbiota results in intestinal inflammation with breaches in the mucosal barrier, allowing bacterial components to gain access to the blood and liver. In other settings, breaching the intestinal barrier has been shown to allow the adjuvant bacterial lipopolysaccharide (LPS) and other bacterial products to escape the gut, so there is precedent for such a process. Now, the first set of pattern recognition receptors come into play. The toll-like receptors TLR4, which is the PRR for LPS, and TLR9, which recognizes bacterial DNA sequences, appear to be the culprits since mice that are genetically defective in either TLR do not develop heightened susceptibility to fatty liver when housed with genetically susceptible mice, even when they harbor a microbiota that would normally promote this disorder. Two sets of PAMPs (LPS and bacterial DNA), one reactive with TLR4, the other with TLR9, are logical candidates to enter the blood from an inflamed intestine. The consequence of sensing microbial products in the liver is the production of TNFα, which is known to be an inducer of fatty liver.

Thus, microbial sensing, IL-18 production, altered intestinal microbiota, gut inflammation, entry of microbial products into the liver, a second round of microbial sensing, and the production of pro-inflammatory cytokines are linked to major metabolic diseases in a way that one would not have even guessed at even a few years ago. Even more remarkably, the inflammasome-based microbial sensing and the attendant production of

IL-18 *diminish* susceptibility to fatty liver while microbial products that enter the blood and are sensed by TLRs in the liver *increase* susceptibility. The striking chain of events illustrates how critical a finely balanced innate immune system is for many aspects of human health.

In other settings, abnormalities in innate immunity and inflammation pathways are associated with major increases in susceptibility to cancer. It has long been known that patients with ulcerative colitis and Crohn's disease have an increased risk of intestinal cancer. Fiona Powrie and her colleagues at Oxford University, using a mouse model system in which there are no cells of the adaptive immune system, showed that infection with the bacterium *Helicobacter hepaticus*[2] markedly increases colonic inflammation and the risk of colon cancer. They observed an increase in the numbers of a cell population called *innate lymphoid cells* (ILCs). The ILCs that accumulate in the colon produce two signature cytokines, IL-17 and IL-22. Blocking IL-22, but not IL-17, by administering an anti-IL-22 antibody reduced both colonic inflammation and colon cancer in these mice, implying a causal link between the innate immune system, inflammation of the colon, and the development of colon cancer. We have just begun to appreciate the importance of a well-controlled innate immune system to health and the panoply of severe consequences to health when the innate system is dysregulated.

23

Evolution of the Immune System and Innate Lymphoid Cells

As we have seen, fruit flies and other invertebrates have an innate immune system but lack the adaptive immune system that consists of lymphocytes and antibodies. The adaptive immune system is critical to humans. Children born with severe defects in the adaptive immune system will not survive unless they receive a bone marrow transplant. To repeat, the innate system is sufficient for invertebrates to survive but not for vertebrates. This suggests that with the appearance of the adaptive immune system, vertebrates shed some aspects of innate immunity. Indeed, analysis of the sea urchin genome indicates that it has more than two hundred toll-like-receptor-related genes, whereas humans have only ten, implying that invertebrates have a much more robust innate immune system than we do.

We may ask what was the selective advantage of the adaptive immune system that led to its appearance and its dominance in vertebrates? It is not simply that the adaptive immune system is necessary for a long and healthy life and that the innate system is adequate only for short-lived creatures. Lobsters are believed to be able to attain great age. George, a lobster caught off Newfoundland in 2008, was estimated to be 140 years old. Some invertebrates obviously can survive for long periods and thus their innate immune systems must be adequate to deal with the many infectious challenges they face living in the wild.

To our knowledge, no invertebrate has an adaptive immune system, but all living vertebrates do. What advantage did the adaptive system provide that it has been taken up and retained over the hundreds of millions of years since the appearance of vertebrates? I do not have an answer to this question although I have always harbored the suspicion that the adaptive system was more efficient. That is, the innate system works by turning loose the mechanisms of inflammation, which almost certainly comes at a great cost in energy expenditure and probably causes much "collateral damage" to tissues of the host, since the innate system cannot effectively target its effector functions to destroy foreign tissue and spare host tissue.

By contrast, the adaptive system allows the selection of a small group of cells that have receptors specific for antigens of the potential pathogen and the response made is to a large degree limited to the expansion and differentiation of those cells. Further, the T and B cell receptors and, most particularly, antibody attack their targets with great precision based on their exquisite specificity, thus limiting collateral damage.

Jawless Vertebrates Have a Different Adaptive Immune System

In 2004, Zeev Pancer and Max Cooper, then at the University of Alabama School of Medicine, made a most remarkable discovery. While many experiments had demonstrated that all jawed vertebrates that had been studied have an adaptive immune response, lampreys and hagfish, the two surviving species of jawless vertebrates (agnathans), had not been shown to have an adaptive immune system. Cooper and Jan Klein, a leading immunogeneticist, became interested in this problem and observed that lampreys had cells that appeared by several criteria to be lymphocytes.

Jawed and jawless vertebrates diverged from a common progenitor about 700 million years ago. The finding of lymphocytes in the jawless vertebrates would suggest the presence of an adaptive immune system. But what type of immune system, if any, do the jawless vertebrates have? Pancer and Cooper could not find any trace of immunoglobulin or T-cell receptor genes, nor do these animals have the genes for the proteins that mediate the recombination events required to form T-cell receptors and immunoglobulins. Earlier work had shown that they lacked MHC genes, so the building blocks of the adaptive immune system of the jawed vertebrates were absent from these animals.

However, in their search of the lamprey genome, Pancer and Cooper identified a large set of genes that went through a rearrangement process to generate mature genes that encode receptor-like molecules. In immunized lampreys, these molecules could be secreted and were shown to bind the immunogen with great specificity. However, in complete contrast to the immune system of the jawed vertebrates, which is based on molecules that are part of what is called the *immunoglobulin super-gene* family, the receptor-like molecules of the lamprey were derived from a totally different protein family. The lamprey's receptors are proteins that contain repeats of leucine-rich sequences—*leucine-rich repeats* (LRRs)—as their structural basis. Detailed analysis showed that the lamprey could develop a vast array of distinct receptors containing highly variable LRR elements, designated *variable lymphocyte receptors* (VLRs), flanked by more conserved LRRs.

Cooper and his colleagues also found that there were at least two different classes of VLRs in lampreys. They found one set on cells and secreted into the blood, resembling antibodies. Another set was confined to the cell membrane and resembled TCRs but, of course, had no chemical relationship whatever to BCRs or TCRs.

The remarkable discovery that two different adaptive immune systems had evolved at a very early stage in vertebrate history strongly implies that the selective advantage of adaptive immunity was very great. It is also a noteworthy example of convergent evolution, since in both types of vertebrates there appear to be T cells and B cells but with entirely unrelated receptors.

Innate Lymphoid Cells: NK Cells

Although the adaptive immune systems of jawed and jawless vertebrates entail entirely different biochemistries, both groups of animals have lymphocytes. The analysis of the expressed genes indicates that they are not merely cells that look like each other but really cells of the same type. This implies that the "first vertebrates," which gave rise to both the jawed and jawless vertebrates, also had lymphocytes, although this cannot be proven since no example of such a primitive animal exists today. Almost certainly, the progenitor of both sets of modern vertebrates lacked an adaptive immune system, as jawed vertebrates have no evidence of genes for the VLRs and jawless vertebrates lack any trace of genes for TCRs or BCRs. If either of the two adaptive systems had been in the common progenitor, then we would expect to see a genetic trace in the sequenced genomes from both sets of descendants. This absence implies that the two adaptive systems developed after the jawed and jawless vertebrates evolved from their common ancestor. Therefore, lymphocytes must have existed before the adaptive immune system. If they did exist but lacked BCRs and TCRs, however, what did they do?

I can make an informed guess about their function because there are modern examples of lymphocytes that lack both BCRs and TCRs. These are the innate lymphoid cells (ILCs). One example of an ILC has been known since the mid-1970s. This cell was detected because it had the ability to kill certain tumor cells and virus-infected cells although it lacked BCRs and TCRs. Because of this apparent *natural killer* activity, it was designated an NK cell. The recognition systems used by NK cells would have been judged by Alice (in Wonderland) as "curioser and curioser."

Although NK cells lack BCRs and TCRs, they do have cell surface receptors. In general, each NK cell has two different types of receptors, one activating, the other inhibitory. The inhibitory receptors are usually specific for major histocompatibility complex molecules. When NK cells encounter a cell expressing the MHC molecules for which their inhibitory receptors are specific, the stimulation of the inhibitory receptor prevents the NK cell from turning on its killer mechanisms. Because most cells of the body have MHC molecules, NK cells are normally maintained in an inactive state.

What would be the value of such a cell and why use such a system? Klaus Karre had the brilliant inspiration that the goal of the NK cell was to detect cells that *lacked* MHC molecules.[1] They recognized "missing self," that is, because their inhibitory receptors were specific for self-MHC molecules, they could be best activated if the MHC molecules of the potential target cells (their "self") were "missing." Why would this be useful?

In many virus-infected cells, the virus has essentially hijacked the protein-synthesizing machinery of the cell and suppressed the production of many normal cellular proteins while causing the cell to produce copious amounts of viral proteins. Killer T cells are a major host response to viral infection. Their TCRs recognize viral peptides loaded into class I MHC molecules. Thus, preferential suppression of MHC molecule synthesis would protect a virus-infected cell against destruction by the killer T cell. The NK cell is the body's strategic response to this virus-induced escape from killer T cells. Cells that lose or markedly diminish their expression of MHC molecules will fail to suppress NK cells. Since NK cells, like killer T cells, can lyse their target cells, the virus-infected cell now could come under attack by the NK cell.

A similar situation exists for tumor cells. Many tumors express new proteins, called *tumor antigens*. Because these antigens are foreign as far as the immune system is concerned, they are, in principle, subject to attack by killer T cells. Tumor cells in which mutations occur that diminish MHC expression (this is actually seen quite often) could therefore escape the killer T cells but would come under attack by NK cells since their lack of MHC molecules would mean they would no longer suppress NK cells.

But this is only part of the story. The NK cell receptor for MHC molecules generally leads to the inactivation of the NK cell. When that receptor is no longer occupied, if MHC molecules are poorly expressed on the virus-infected cell or the tumor cell, the NK cell is no longer actively suppressed. But the NK cell has a second receptor, often referred to as an *activating receptor*. NK cell activating receptors generally recognize a class of molecules expressed by cells under stress. Viral infection or malignant transformation are interpreted by a cell as stressors and accordingly, these cells express cell surface molecules that the NK cell's activating receptor can recognize. Thus, the combination of lack of restraint by the inhibitory receptor and activation by the activating receptor makes the NK cell a formidable bodily weapon against virally infected cells and certain tumor cells.

ILC 1, 2, and 3 Cells

NK cells were well known and actively studied since the 1970s. However, not until recently did researchers identify other cell types that also lacked BCRs and TCRs, were lymphocyte in appearance, and had effector functions that had been thought of as mainly characteristic of T cells. These are the cells designated ILCs.

The NK cell engages in killer activity but can also make cytokines, particularly IFNγ. Moreover, the NK cell can be stimulated to make these cytokines not only through the engagement of its activating receptor but also when it is stimulated by certain other cytokines. The most efficient *cytokine-induced cytokine production* by NK cells utilizes two stimulatory cytokines, IL-12 and IL-18.

The ability of a combination of two cytokines, both representing a distinct class of activators, to cause NK cells to make cytokines turns out to be shared, to a greater or lesser degree, by ILCs. IL-12 is a member of a class of cytokines that causes the activation of a particular biochemical pathway in its target cells. The key element of that pathway is a member of a set of signal transducing and transactivating (STAT) molecules. Once activated, the STATs enter the nucleus, target a specific set of genes, and aid in their activation so that they now transcribe mRNA, leading to the production of a new set of proteins. There are seven distinct STATs. Different cytokines activate different STATs, and each STAT has a specific set of target genes, establishing a connection between the stimulating cytokine and the proteins that are produced. IL-12 activates STAT4; STAT4 plays an important role in the production of IFNγ.

IL-18 is a member of the interleukin-1 family of molecules of which the index member is IL-1. The members of this family are similar to each other in their overall structure; their receptors have a substantial degree of similarity and, as we saw for IL-1β, they activate NF-κB, which plays an important role in cytokine production. Different cell types are characterized by having receptors for different members of the IL-1 family.

ILC2 cells have some resemblance to Th2 cells, which have been shown to be very important in immunity to a class of parasitic worms called helminths, including hookworm and schistosomes (see chapter 17). While we in the western world have largely eliminated these as threats, they remain a major health concern in many parts of the developing world.

A favorite experimental system through which to study the biology of protective immunity to helminths is to infect mice with the larvae of *Nippostrongylus brasiliensis*, a parasite that resembles hookworm. The larvae migrate from the site of injection, usually the skin, into the mouse's lungs and are then coughed up by the mouse and enter the intestine where they develop into mature worms and begin to lay eggs that will then be passed out in the feces.

Mice make a vigorous adaptive immune response to "Nippo" so that by days eleven to thirteen after infection, all the worms are expelled. The key to the expulsion of the worms is the action of the cytokine IL-13. IL-13 has many functions but an important one is to stimulate the intestinal musculature to force the worms out. IL-13 is closely related to IL-4, the cytokine Maureen Howard and I discovered. Among T cells, IL-13 is made principally by Th2 cells. It is known that T cells are essential to the expulsion of the parasite as is IL-13, and there is good evidence that Th2 cells play a critical role.

Careful study of mice infected with Nippo showed that many of the IL-13-producing cells that appear, while lymphocyte like in appearance and in many of the genes they express, lacked the critical markers associated with T cells. They did not express CD4, CD8, or the TCR. Neither were they other types of lymphocytes, such as B cells. They did express the receptor for an IL-1 family member, IL-33, and they made as much or more IL-13 per cell than did Th2 cells.

Although ILC2 cells could be easily detected in mice that had been infected with Nippo or in mice treated with IL-33, in normal mice the numbers of these cells were very small. But mice that lack these cells, as a result of the disruption of a gene whose product is critical for their development, show a very substantial delay in the expulsion of Nippo. Thus, ILC2 cells are innate cells (they lacked BCRs and TCRs), they are lymphoid (lymphocyte like), and they make many of the cytokines that Th2 cells made, hence the name ILC2. It appears the early innate responses made by ILC2 cells, while not able to eliminate a parasite by themselves (mice without T cells cannot eliminate Nippo), play a critical early role in immunity. Without them, resistance to helminths is markedly diminished.

ILC2 cells express the receptor for the IL-1 homolog IL-33, and injecting IL-33 into mice causes an increase in their numbers. IL-33 treatment also causes these cells to make IL-13 and this production is increased if they are treated at the same time with a cytokine that activates STAT5. That molecule is known as thymic stromal lymphopoietin (TSLP). Activated STAT5 is known to directly target the IL-13 gene so that the combination of NF-κB induction by IL-33 and targeting of the IL-13 gene by TSLP leads to robust production of IL-13.

ILC1 and ILC3 cells also contribute to infection resistance, acting early, before the adaptive response has "geared up." In situations in which cells of the adaptive system are not available, ILCs can sometimes be effective in resisting infection. ILC1 cells, like Th1 cells, produce IFNγ and use the transcription factor T-bet. ILC3 cells resemble Th17 and Th22 cells in terms of the cytokines they produce and the transcription factors they express.

Although we cannot be certain in the absence of any living representative of the most primitive vertebrates, it is a good bet that they used ILCs or ILC-like cells to protect against infection. It is interesting to speculate whether they had already achieved the specialization of modern ILCs (i.e., into ILC1, ILC2, ILC3, and NK cells). Such a specialization would have been valuable as it would have allowed these primitive vertebrates to develop "appropriate" responses—ILC1 for viruses and intracellular bacteria, ILC2 for helminths, and ILC3 for extracellular bacteria—even in the absence of adaptive immunity.

VI AIDS, AUTOIMMUNITY, ALLERGY, CANCER, AND TRANSPLANTATION

The HIV Epidemic and the Office of AIDS Research

AIDS burst on the scene in the early 1980s with devastating effects on at-risk populations, including gay men, intravenous drug users, and recipients of blood products, such as people who have hemophilia. To those in the affected groups, it appeared that nearly all their friends were afflicted with this terrible infection; many were dying dreadful deaths. Although the fact that the gay community was more affected than other groups may have slowed the response by some in government, there can be little doubt that the world research community rose to the effort to combat this completely unanticipated threat. Funding by the National Institutes of Health, which provides the vast majority of money for biomedical research in the United States, revved up slowly at first but then rose exponentially so that by 1993 it exceeded $1.3 billion.

Nonetheless, the AIDS advocacy community grew increasingly desperate and was not convinced that NIH was attacking the AIDS problem in an effective manner. Various activist groups appeared, of which ACT-UP New York was perhaps the best known. By 1992, some in the community were becoming concerned about the effectiveness of ACT-UP's strategy of confrontation and had come to the conclusion that the surest way to make progress against AIDS was to work for a greater scientific attack on the root causes of the disease.

Members of ACT-UP New York left and formed the Treatment Action Group (TAG) in 1992 to martial advocates' efforts to promote research on AIDS and HIV. TAG's members and others in the advocacy community lobbied Congress very effectively, arguing that AIDS research money was being poorly spent and that to be effective, there needed to be a central decision-making process that would insure AIDS research money was effectively targeted.

In the NIH Revitalization Act of 1993, Congress designated a new role for the NIH Office of AIDS Research (OAR). Until then, the OAR had been a relatively obscure entity in the NIH Director's Office that helped to coordinate the AIDS research programs of the various institutes of NIH and reported on how resources were being used. Now, Congress was mandating that the office "have the authority to plan, coordinate, and evaluate AIDS research, to set scientific priorities, and to determine the budgets for all NIH Institute and Center AIDS research."[1] This directive was close to anathema to the NIH leadership. It would remove the power for planning the research effort from the individual institutes, including the National Institute of Allergy and Infectious Diseases and the National Cancer Institute, the two institutes with the largest portfolio of grants and contracts aimed at HIV and AIDS, and transfer it to some central authority. Also, it would lead to centrally planned research, which the NIH leaders believed, with some justice, was as likely to be successful in controlling HIV as central economic planning had been in the Soviet Union. Despite NIH opposition, the Congress gave the OAR the responsibility of developing an overarching plan for AIDS research. All funds for NIH-sponsored AIDS research were to be allocated to the OAR, which would then distribute them to the institutes to use in a manner in accord with the central plan.

Once the NIH Revitalization Act was passed, the NIH was faced with responding to the congressional directive. This fell to director Harold Varmus to accomplish. A world-renowned scientist, Varmus had studied the class of viruses known as retroviruses, of which HIV is a member. These viruses received their name because their genome is made of single-stranded RNA. In infected cells, this single-stranded RNA acts as a template on which DNA that is a complementary copy of the RNA is formed and which then incorporates into the genome of the host cell, thereafter acting as a cellular gene, although a highly unusual one. In typical cells, genetic information is stored in DNA, and RNA (messenger RNA) is the intermediate toward the production of the protein products of the gene. Since the genetic information flow is reversed in viruses with single-stranded-RNA genomes, the viruses are "retroviruses."

Varmus and his colleague Michael Bishop at the University of California, San Francisco, had carried out a remarkable series of studies that identified the origin of retroviruses' oncogenes, which helped to cause cells infected with these viruses to become malignant. Bishop and Varmus showed that oncogenes had originally been cellular genes that the viruses had hijacked and that the genes had mutated so that they now instructed the infected cell to undergo unregulated growth and acquire other characteristics of tumor cells. They received the 1989 Nobel Prize in Physiology or Medicine for this work. Varmus had been at NIH from 1968 to 1970 as a commissioned officer in the US Public Health Service, fulfilling his military obligation. He was one of the nine NIH postdocs in that golden era who later won Nobel Prizes.

The congressional mandate for the expanded role of the OAR came at a time when the AIDS advocacy community was in a state of deep gloom. There had just been an international AIDS conference in Berlin. No breakthroughs had been announced at the conference, and it appeared that little was being accomplished. That was actually not true; in fact, the next several years would see remarkable advances powered by work that had been done in 1993 and before. But superficially, it looked as if the research effort were going nowhere.

Bernard Fields, the chairman of the Department of Microbiology and Molecular Genetics at Harvard Medical School, wrote a very influential op-ed in the highly respected scientific journal *Nature* in which he called for a "back to basics" approach for AIDS research.[2] Success, he argued, was as likely to arise from unrelated areas of research as from an AIDS-directed research program. Fields's position would seem to be the antithesis of the centralization of planning for AIDS research through the OAR, but paradoxically the message encouraged strong support of the OAR process.

Harold Varmus appointed a search committee for the OAR director. I was asked to serve on the committee as a scientist with a deep knowledge of basic immunology. We made major efforts to encourage qualified AIDS researchers to apply for the position, but the deep politicalization of the process may well have discouraged potential candidates. We were left with applications from good but not truly outstanding individuals, with one major exception. Bernie Fields had submitted an application. He appeared before the search committee and it was clear that he was exceptionally qualified for the position. The committee was unanimous that he would make a first-rate OAR director.

There was one issue, however. Bernie had been diagnosed with pancreatic cancer, and the disease was now in remission. Indeed, he said that his enthusiasm to undertake the challenge of being OAR director was to a degree predicated on "his getting his life back." He told the committee that if he were offered the position, he would accept it. However, he was scheduled to have a CAT scan that he hoped would show he was still cancer-free. Unfortunately, the scan revealed that he had had a recurrence, which effectively meant he could not take on the directorship. Bernie continued to do his utmost to promote a program of high-quality scientific research in AIDS; meanwhile, the cancer progressed, and he died in January 1995.

Harold Varmus was left in a difficult position. His one truly outstanding candidate for the Office of AIDS Research directorship was unavailable. In the fall of 1993, he called me into his office in Building 1 on the NIH campus and asked me to take on the responsibility. I was taken aback. Although I had followed the HIV/AIDS field and of course knew the immunological issues, I had never worked on the disease or the virus, and I was concerned about dealing with the politics, the advocacy groups, and what was by now a large research budget.

Marilyn and I discussed these issues at length, and I sought advice from colleagues, in particular Anthony Fauci, who was director of the National Institute of Allergy and Infectious Diseases and one of the world's preeminent AIDS researchers. I knew Tony quite well, not least because his research group and mine had held joint lab meetings during the period we were working on IL-4 and he was studying a human cytokine that was important in B-cell function.

In the end, I concluded that I had to take on the responsibility. The AIDS epidemic was such that one really didn't have a choice. Even though I realized my preparation to be OAR director might be less than ideal, it was clear that this position would be extremely important for the progress of research in the field, and I felt sure that I would come to the position with no axes to grind.

Accordingly, I resigned from the search committee, submitted an application, and was offered the position. It was essential that the Office of AIDS Research get off to a running start to demonstrate to the world that it intended to fulfill its responsibility and to do so in a way that would promote the highest standard of research, not threaten it. I was sensitive to a perception by some that though scientifically qualified for the position, I might not be willing to take a vigorous leadership position particularly if I received pushback from the NIH leadership, many of whom were friends.

Within the first week or two after my appointment, I convened a meeting at Stone House on the NIH campus of some of the leading virologists, immunologists, molecular biologists, and AIDS researchers, including David Baltimore, a discoverer of the RNA to DNA pathway used by retroviruses; Phil Sharp, who had discovered that genes were not continuous and that a process of splicing was important in the production of messenger RNA; Harold Varmus; and several others.

From the Stone House meeting, I came away with the clear need to pursue a comprehensive review of all NIH-sponsored AIDS research, which would prove to be a truly vast undertaking. This review needed to be done by an outside group of scientists, with OAR acting as staff. I persuaded Arnold Levine, chairman of the Department of Molecular Biology at Princeton, later president of the Rockefeller University, and now a professor emeritus at the Institute for Advanced Study, to take on this task. Arnie had discovered p53, one of the key proteins that regulate cellular growth and that is deranged in cancer. He had an encyclopedic knowledge of cancer and virology as well as being indefatigable and a highly effective organizer.

Arnie attacked this problem with vigor and my colleague in the OAR, Bob Eisinger, acted as his principal staffer. The Levine report, when it appeared, became the basic document for all subsequent AIDS research and validated the OAR approach.[3] However, before that report could be issued, we needed to organize the planning process, establish priorities, give the NIH institutes guidance for the preparation of their research programs, and then develop a coordinated budget built according to the research plan. I was determined that while the planning process had to represent the best thinking in the field, it could not be too proscriptive. We didn't want to quash creativity, without which progress was sure to be hampered.

I was fortunate in that treatment advances began to occur that started to dispel the gloom that had pervaded the advocacy and scientific communities. Shortly after I became OAR director, it was reported that the transmission of HIV infection from mothers to their newborns could be effectively prevented by treatment of the mother during pregnancy and the newborn with the drugs available at the time, which were blockers of the action of the enzyme necessary to copy RNA into DNA.[4] The best known of these drugs was AZT. Effectively, it meant that we could prevent almost all babies born in the United States from being infected from their mothers.

This was the first of the successes that transformed the view of the advocacy communities and convinced them that science was the answer. Although the OAR and I had had nothing to do with this work, it led to a validation of the OAR process. As the principal representative of the AIDS research effort, our position with Congress and the advocacy community was immeasurably strengthened.

Shortly afterward, a new class of drugs to treat HIV infection was introduced, the protease inhibitors. These proved extremely effective and had a transforming effect on treatment. When the protease inhibitors were used in combination with the older drugs, the likelihood that resistant virus would appear was markedly diminished. Indeed, the optimism generated was such that the treatment was called *highly active antiretroviral therapy* (HAART). After the introduction of HAART, I was seated at dinner with Mark Harrington, one of the founders of TAG and a recipient of a MacArthur "genius" award. Mark turned to me and said that he had started to contribute to his individual retirement account. The change in attitude in just a few years was immensely gratifying.

While the introduction of HAART brightened the prospects for those infected with HIV, the rate of new infections was not declining. During my tenure at the OAR, it remained at around 40,000 new cases per year in the United States. The situation in areas of high prevalence such as sub-Saharan Africa was far worse.

Let's review what we knew about the course of the infection and the onset of AIDS. Infection occurred through unprotected sex, intravenous drug use, or receipt of blood products that contained virus. Fortunately, with the development of good tests for HIV, the blood supply had been made safe, as were the blood products used to treat patients with hemophilia.

Infected individuals would begin with a systemwide infection affecting many of their CD4 T cells. This was particularly notable in the intestine, where a large proportion of the CD4 T cells became infected and died. The virus particularly targeted Th17 cells, which help maintain the mucosal barrier. Most of the infected cells died, but not before they had produced more virus and infected other cells. Furthermore, some of the infected cells, rather than dying, reverted to a resting state, with the HIV genome copied into their cellular genes but remaining inactive. These cells are regarded as having been *latently infected* and essentially invisible to the immune system. They represent a potential source of virus when (or if) they became reactivated. Indeed, the presence of this long-lived reservoir of HIV in latently infected cells is the major impediment to the eradication of HIV.

The HIV-mediated killing of CD4 T cells in the intestine resulted in a breach in the mucosal barrier and the entry of bacterial products into the blood, causing a state of inflammation. The amount of virus in the blood peaks shortly after infection. It falls dramatically and remains relatively low for a very long time, perhaps ten years. Although "viral burden" is low during this period, excess inflammation continues, possibly because the depletion of gut CD4 T cells is not fully repaired even when the virus is controlled by drugs. The current view is that the continuing inflammatory response seen in HIV-infected persons plays a central role in the gradual loss of immune function in untreated individuals and their eventual progression to AIDS. The degree of inflammation may be a better predictor of prognosis than the amount of virus or the number of CD4 T cells found in the blood.

The onset of AIDS is defined by the fall in the number of CD4 T cells in the blood below 200 per cubic millimeter, with the normal counts in adults being 500 to 1,000; by the appearance of one of a set of opportunistic infections; or by the development of certain cancers, such as Kaposi's sarcoma or lymphomas. With the onset of AIDS, the amount of virus increases precipitously. Antiretroviral therapy has allowed us to prevent or markedly delay progression to AIDS in the majority of patients and thus has had an enormous impact on the prognosis of infected individuals.

But while treating HIV infection adequately represents a great step forward, what would be an even greater breakthrough would be a way to eradicate HIV from the body (a cure) or a way to prevent infection. During my period in the Office of AIDS Research, I was particularly anxious to make progress toward a preventive vaccine.

I took the OAR position in February 1994 and developed a centralized plan of HIV research, using the expertise of a wide range of scientists and members of the advocacy community and with the support of key members of the OAR, particularly deputy director Jack Whitescarver and Wendy Wertheimer, my senior adviser.

Our goal was to allow substantial flexibility but to guide the research to what we viewed as the most productive and important areas. However, I was convinced that we should do our utmost to encourage the creativity of the scientific community so I made it a priority that the institutes move away from a heavy reliance on contracts and other mechanisms through which those at NIH called the shots. I strongly encouraged a shift toward research project grants in which scientists would prepare research proposals and submit them for review by panels of independent scientists (study sections), with those receiving the highest priority being funded. This strategy was clearly bearing fruit.

In the fall of 1996, I had been in the Office of AIDS Research for almost three years. I was deeply concerned that progress toward developing a preventive vaccine for HIV had been very slow. I thought it essential that we make vaccine research a priority and in the annual plan then under development, we shifted substantial resources to HIV vaccine research. Then, a unique opportunity presented itself on December 1, 1996.

December 1 is World AIDS Day. President Clinton invited Harold Varmus, Tony Fauci, and me from NIH, and Helene Gayle from the CDC to the White House to brief him on the current status of efforts against the disease. HAART was showing its great effectiveness, and Tony Fauci and the others emphasized drug treatment of disease. I resolved that my "pitch" would be that we needed to invest heavily in vaccine research. When we reached the Oval Office, we were told that the president was running late, and since I was to be the last to speak, I might very well not have my opportunity. Fate intervened and I did get my few minutes during which I emphasized the critical need for a protective vaccine. I had made a similar point to the president when he had visited NIH earlier, but this time, I must have struck a responsive chord.

I had formulated, with the very significant help of Ron Germain, my colleague in the Laboratory of Immunology, the plan of developing an HIV vaccine research center (VRC) at NIH. Harold Varmus and Tony Fauci were strong supporters of this concept, and we were able to get buy-in from the chairs of the Senate and House Appropriations Sub-Committees, Arlen Spector and John Porter.

An appropriation to establish the VRC on the NIH campus was included in the budget. However, the amount allocated was somewhat less than required to build the type of research building we thought necessary. Fortunately, the OAR had been receiving royalties that had come as a result of the joint agreement between the French and American governments about the HIV blood test. Unlike government-appropriated funds that could not be carried over from year to year, these royalty funds could be saved. I was able to add $7 million to the building fund, assuring that a first-rate research building could be built to house the VRC. The Dale and Betty Bumpers Vaccine Research Center was dedicated in 1998.

Having brought the VRC to fruition and increased the resources devoted to HIV vaccine research, as well as presiding over a period of substantial scientific and medical progress, I decided that my term at the OAR should draw to a close. I was convinced that if I stayed longer as OAR director, it would be almost impossible to reestablish myself as a productive research scientist. So in November 1997, I stepped down from the Office of AIDS Research with a sense of considerable satisfaction but, of course, recognizing how far we still had to go.

25

How the Immune System Causes Rheumatoid Arthritis and Lupus

Failures in tolerance mechanisms can lead to a generalized state of autoimmunity. For example, APECED is a disease that develops because of a defect in clonal deletion. The defect results because of a failure of certain proteins to be manufactured in the mTECs, a specialized cell type in the thymic medulla, thus allowing self-antigen-specific cells to avoid negative selection (see chapter 14). In the disease called IPEX, a mutation in the master regulatory transcription factor of Tregs, Foxp3, results in the failure of Tregs to develop and thus to autoimmunity due to lack of suppression of the activation of self-reactive T cells (see chapter 15).

Serious autoimmune diseases affect many people in the world—usually without a cause that we can discern. Among these are type 1 diabetes mellitus, multiple sclerosis, the inflammatory bowel diseases, myasthenia gravis, scleroderma, thyroiditis, systemic lupus erythematosus, and rheumatoid arthritis. Our understanding of the processes through which these diseases occur is still limited, but in some areas there has been progress. We know a great deal about what the T cells are specific for in type 1 diabetes, the nature of the immune response that destroys the β cells of the islets of Langerhans, and we can often identify children at increased risk of developing type 1 diabetes based on the presence of antibodies to insulin in their blood long before diabetes appears and their being of a particular class II major histocompatibility complex type, HLA/DR3/4. Major efforts are being made to use that information either to forestall development of diabetes or to treat it in the very early stages, before all the patient's insulin-producing cells have been destroyed, but success has been elusive. Nonetheless, knowledge that a child is at risk of developing type 1 diabetes allows parents to be on the lookout for early signs that might be followed by diabetic coma, so that at least that life-threatening event can be avoided.

Multiple sclerosis has also been studied in great detail. The origin of MS is unknown, but its cause is immune-mediated destruction of the cells that produce the myelin sheath, which coats the projections of the nerve cells, the axons. In the absence of myelin, the transmission of nerve impulses is slowed, thus impairing the connections between the cells of the nervous system and disrupting nerve function. The disease appears, in many cases, episodic, with severe progressive events followed by some degree of recovery. However, analysis of the brain with modern imaging technology suggests a more continuing progression.

The most exciting advance in the effort to treat multiple sclerosis is the introduction of monoclonal antibodies that block the pathway through which T cells may enter the brain. In order to enter the brain, T lymphocytes use a cell surface molecule, designated an *integrin*. The integrin interacts with a specific type of adhesion molecule, allowing the cells to pass through the lining layer of the blood vessels and gain entry to the brain itself. A monoclonal antibody, *nataluzimab*, specific for a component of that integrin, has proven quite effective in the treatment of multiple sclerosis, presumably because it blocks entry of disease-inducing lymphocytes into the brain.

One side effect is that nataluzimab also blocks the entry of lymphocytes that provide protection against infection with a particular virus, the JC virus, which can cause a potentially fatal neurological condition, *progressive multifocal leukoencephalopathy* (PML). When natalizumab was initially introduced, a few cases of PML appeared, leading to withdrawal of the drug from the market. However, with suitable precautions, mainly testing patients for antibodies to the JC virus as evidence of infection and taking patients off treatment if increased amounts of the antibodies are observed, the drug has been successfully reintroduced.

Several experimental models in mice have been helpful in understanding how the lesions in MS occur. In general, these models consist of immunizing mice with proteins isolated from the myelin sheath, mainly myelin basic protein (MBP) or myelin oligodendrocyte glycoprotein (MOG), together with complete Freund's adjuvant. Immunized animals of susceptible inbred strains develop experimental allergic encephalomyelitis (EAE). EAE is marked mainly by paralysis to varying degrees of the tail and the hind limbs. It is mainly due to the development of Th1 or Th17 CD4 T cells specific for MBP or MOG. It appears that both cell types are important in the induction and progression of the disease, and eliminating either cell type through genetic engineering or other methods prevents or markedly diminishes the disease.

Let's look more closely at two autoimmune diseases, rheumatoid arthritis (RA) and systemic lupus erythematosus (SLE), as they illustrate both the conundrums still facing the scientific and medical communities and how our growing understanding of immune responses has led to advances in treatment.

Rheumatoid Arthritis

RA is an inflammatory disease with systemwide effects. The major abnormalities are in the joints and surrounding tissues. Each joint in the human body is enclosed within a synovial sac. In RA, there is marked synovial inflammation, with the presence of large numbers of inflammatory cells and increased fluid within the joint space, and the deposition of fibrous tissue. As the disease progresses, the cartilage that lines the surfaces of the bones that are articulated in a joint is progressively destroyed, and there is often loss of bone. People with progressive disease can have severe joint deformities and major loss of function.

There are many reasons to believe that RA is due to a lymphocyte response to antigens of tissues within the joint, although much of the actual tissue damage is due to the consequent inflammatory response that develops in the joint. Like many autoimmune diseases, the most important genetic factor that predisposes to developing RA is an HLA[1] gene, in this case HLA-DR4. In one study, individuals who were HLA-DR4+ were ten times more likely to develop RA than were DR4− individuals. One possibility to explain this increased likelihood is that HLA-DR4 acts as an Ir gene that is permissive for the development of an immune response to some critical, but still unknown, antigen that plays a role in the development of RA.

Antibodies to citrulline[2] in peptides are found in the great majority of people with RA and may be detected two years or more before the onset of clinical disease. Whether these antibodies to citrullinated peptides contribute to the development of arthritis or are simply markers of the immune response that causes the disease is still uncertain. However, in experimental models of RA, antibodies often play an important role in the development of the inflammatory state.

There are several mouse models of induced arthritis with features that resemble rheumatoid arthritis. The most widely studied is *collagen-induced arthritis* (CIA). CIA results from immunizing genetically susceptible strains of mice with type II collagen and complete Freund's adjuvant. Collagen is a protein that is the principal component of fibrous tissue; type II collagen is found particularly in cartilage. Type II collagen–immunized mice rapidly develop a severe arthritis in which the abnormalities in the joints resemble those of RA in humans.

The susceptibility of some strains of mice to CIA and the resistance of others is due, at least in part, to the MHC alleles the mice possess. As I already proposed for RA, the role of MHC in determining susceptibility to CIA strongly suggests that T cells play a major role in the induction of the disease. However, in contrast to many other autoimmune diseases, antibodies, here to type II collagen, are critical to the progression of CIA. Mice that are unable to produce antibodies because of a genetically engineered deletion in genes necessary for antibody production are protected against CIA.

Treatment for RA had stagnated for many years. The most effective treatment had been use of low doses of methotrexate. Methotrexate was the drug that led to cure of choriocarcinoma (see chapter 4). The doses of methotrexate for treatment of RA and choriocarcinoma are very different. How methotrexate acts to control RA is unknown. But a breakthrough in RA treatment came with the recognition that inflammatory cytokines, such as TNFα, were responsible for much of the tissue damage and that by blocking these cytokines, the disease could be ameliorated. The contributions of two individuals stand out in the process of introducing monoclonal anti-TNFα antibody for the treatment of RA. They are Marc Feldmann and Ravinder Maini, a basic immunologist and an RA clinician.

Feldmann was born in Lvov, Poland, in 1944. After the war, his family managed to get to France and then emigrated to Australia when Marc was eight. Marc received his medical education in Melbourne and earned a PhD at the Walter and Eliza Hall Institute in Melbourne (an institute that is a recurring presence in this book). After completing his PhD, Marc came to the UK to do a postdoc under the supervision of Av Mitchison, who had by then moved to University College London to occupy the same chair that his mentor, Peter Medawar, had held. Marc spent his early years in London as a basic immunologist, working on lymphocyte biology. But he became increasingly interested in autoimmune diseases and wished to understand how the immune system mediated the severe tissue damage that was the hallmark of these diseases.

After an effort to study thyroiditis, he turned to what he considered a more tractable problem, RA. In 1984, he began a collaboration with Ravinder Maini. Maini was a leading RA clinician and student of the pathogenesis of the disease. He was born in the Punjab region of India but had lived most of his life in the UK. Educated in Cambridge, Maini was associated with the Kennedy Institute of Rheumatology in London, where he became director. Ravinder Maini, not a man of short stature, was nonetheless widely known as "Tiny" and when he was later knighted for his work on RA, some referred to him as Sir Tiny.

Feldmann and Maini instituted a set of studies aimed at understanding the immunologic and inflammatory abnormalities in RA. They established that macrophages from the synovial fluid of persons with RA overproduced TNFα and other pro-inflammatory cytokines. They then showed that antibodies to TNFα diminished the production of other pro-inflammatory cytokines by synovial cells from people with rheumatoid arthritis. This led them to the concept that TNFα was the "top" cytokine in an inflammation cascade. They reasoned that if they could block TNFα, they might halt the inflammation that was at the heart of disease progression in RA. Feldmann and Maini first showed that administering an antibody to TNFα to mice that were immunized with type II collagen would block the onset of CIA. This finding strengthened their idea that TNFα was central to the development or progression of RA.

Feldmann and Maini were then resolved to carry out a clinical trial of the efficacy of anti-human-TNFα in treating RA. A suitable antibody existed. Jan Vilcek, a professor of microbiology at the New York University School of Medicine, had prepared a monoclonal antibody to human TNFα. Initially, it was hoped that such antibodies could be used to treat septic shock, a life-threatening condition, usually the result of severe infection and often associated with high blood levels of pro-inflammatory cytokines such as TNFα. Unfortunately, monoclonal antibodies to TNFα failed to reverse septic shock, and interest in the clinical use of these antibodies had waned.

Vilcek's antibody had been developed by the biotech firm Centocor but was essentially on the shelf. At the time, the chief scientific officer of Centocor was Jim Woody, who had done postdoctoral training with Marc Feldmann. Discussions by Marc and Tiny with Jim and his colleagues at Centocor resulted in the go-ahead for a clinical trial. In the initial trial, anti-TNFα proved to be remarkably successful in preventing progression in RA and a subsequent large phase III international trial confirmed this effect. Vilcek's anti-TNFα became the drug infliximab, which not only was extremely successful as a treatment for RA and other inflammatory conditions but demonstrated to the pharmaceutical industry the great promise of monoclonal antibodies as drugs.

Although the technology had been available for several years, monoclonal antibodies had not been in favor as drugs because they were expensive to make and the market for these agents was not deemed to be sufficient for a major investment. The great success of infliximab led to an almost complete reversal in this view. There are now at least thirty FDA-approved monoclonal antibodies and more on the way.

Feldmann and Maini received many honors for their pioneering work in the treatment of RA. Both were knighted, they shared the Albert and Mary Lasker Foundation Clinical Research Prize, and both were elected as foreign members of the US National Academy of Sciences.

Of course, it should be recognized that anti-TNFα blocks the effector arm of the immune response in RA; it does not inhibit the T-cell response that is at the heart of the disease. The goal remains to understand how T cells become activated and to find a way to reverse the action of these autoimmune T cells or, even better, to predict the likelihood that an individual would develop RA and to develop strategies to prevent the disease.

Thus, RA, while far better treated today than in the pre-anti-TNFα era, is still a major problem. The treatment is expensive; it does not work in every patient (although there are now other monoclonal antibodies targeting other inflammatory cytokines that may be of value in such cases); and its effect is not complete. We need to understand the aberrant T-cell response that initiates the disease and the antibody response that is critical to its progression. Preventing disease onset or reversing the T- or B-cell responses would be a far better solution than blocking the end-stage inflammation. But make no mistake, anti-TNFα has been transformative in treating RA and has set a standard for the treatment of other autoimmune and auto-inflammatory diseases.

Systemic Lupus Erythematosus

SLE is one of the most enigmatic and devastating of the autoimmune diseases. In most other autoimmune diseases, a major organ is the principal target. But SLE is a generalized disease in which virtually every organ system of the body can be affected. It is mainly a disease of women, with onset in the child-bearing years. Often, what brings the patient to her doctor initially is the appearance of a very characteristic butterfly facial rash largely confined to the cheeks (described as a *malar rash*), which actually is responsible for the name of the disease. It was initially thought to have been due to a wolf bite (which seems very difficult to credit). Since *lupus* is the Latin for "wolf," and *erythematosus* implies a reddened rash, *lupus erythematosus* was the designation. It was only in the twentieth century that it was recognized that women with the characteristic rash of lupus had multi-organ autoimmunity and the designation "systemic" was added.

It is generally believed that SLE is due to a generalized failure of normal immune regulation. Its effect on almost every organ system results from the formation of antibodies against many different self-tissues. A particularly characteristic antibody found in the great majority of patients with SLE, but rarely seen in normal individuals, is specific for double-stranded DNA (dsDNA). The presence of anti-dsDNA antibodies is an important criteria in the diagnosis. Almost everyone with clinical signs and symptoms of SLE will have these antibodies in her blood at some time during the disease.

Not only are anti-dsDNA antibodies important in making the diagnosis of SLE, they can be responsible for some of the most severe and life-threatening aspects of the disease. People with lupus have dsDNA in the blood and tissues because of excess death of cells, probably as a result of ongoing cellular apoptosis. Anti-dsDNA antibodies bind to dsDNA and create an "immune complex" consisting of the antibody and antigen. The immune complexes can deposit in the kidneys of patients and lead to severe nephritis that, if untreated, can be fatal.

In addition, the immune complexes that contain dsDNA can stimulate TLR9, one of the human toll-like receptors; dsDNA is the pathogen-associated molecular pattern for the TLR9 pattern recognition receptor. TLR9 is not expressed on the cell surface but rather is found in the cell within lysosomes, which are membrane-bounded structures that fuse with the vacuoles that contain substances brought into the cell by phagocytosis and through the related process of endocytosis. An immune complex consisting of antibodies and dsDNA is an efficient way to target the dsDNA to lysosomal TLR9. The antibody in the complex is bound by specific receptors on macrophages that bind the Fc portion of antibody (Fc receptors). As a result, the complex of anti-dsDNA and dsDNA enters the cell through an endosome, which fuses with a lysosome, and thus the dsDNA gains access to TLR9. This stimulation will cause the macrophage to produce large amounts of type I interferons. Type I interferons, in turn, activate many genes that contribute to the multi-organ inflammation in SLE.

We can be fairly certain this is how SLE proceeds because research groups, beginning with Mary Crow's at the Hospital for Special Surgery in New York City and Virginia Pascual and Jacques Banchereau's, then working at the Baylor Institute for Immunology Research in Dallas, have shown that most people with SLE had a pattern of gene expression in their blood cells that displayed an "interferon signature." In 2003, Pascual and Banchereau reported the results of measuring gene expression profiles in SLE patients. Their results showed that virtually all SLE patients expressed genes known to be turned on by type I interferon to a much greater degree than did normal individuals. This was one of the first and most impressive uses of the new techniques of molecular biology to gain insight to the mechanism through which the abnormalities of a disease are mediated.

SLE, because it affects so many different organs, can have a very different pattern of abnormalities in different people. People with SLE experience frequent flares in their symptomatology, and the flares are unpredictable. These aspects of the disease have made drug companies reluctant to conduct clinical trials in SLE and has almost certainly held back drug development. Until recently, virtually no new drugs had been introduced for SLE. Many patients were maintained on high doses of steroids, with the inevitable toxicity that these potent drugs cause. In addition, patients with nephritis are often treated with cyclophosphamide, azathioprine, or mycophenolate mofetil.

Very recently, belimumab, a monoclonal antibody that inhibits B-cell activating factor (BAFF), a cytokine important in the development of B cells, has been shown to have some effect in controlling SLE and has been approved by the FDA. Nonetheless, there is a clear need for new drugs that can act at the induction stage of SLE and block the progression of the disease. Despite a long history of research, the mechanism through which the disease occurs is poorly understood.

For that reason, a group of family members of people with SLE founded the Lupus Research Institute (LRI) in 2002, with the goal of supporting innovative research, particularly by young scientists and by scientists new to the field of lupus. Their hope was (and continues to be) that creative scientists would bring fresh ideas toward clarifying the cause or causes of SLE and developing new targets for drug development. I was asked to chair the LRI Scientific Advisory Board in 2002, which I continue to do.

LRI has a program of starter grants aimed at bringing highly innovative scientists into the field and getting their projects started, with the hope that they can then become competitive to receive the much larger amounts of funding available from government research funding agencies, particularly from the National Institutes of Health. In that, it has been very successful. Nonetheless, research into SLE has shown how complex this disorder is; we still do not have a true picture of what incites the disease and what controls its progression. But the pharmaceutical and biotech industries have now recognized that modern technologies offer a much greater hope of developing effective therapeutics and guided, in part, by scientific advances funded by the NIH and LRI have made efforts to develop new drugs for SLE a priority.

26

Allergy and Asthma

Hypersensitivities to various pollens are among the most frequent of medical conditions. It has been estimated that around 10 percent of the U.S. population has seasonal allergic rhinitis: runny nose, itchy eyes, and sneezing in response to seasonal allergens. Often the symptoms can be controlled with antihistamines or other medications, but these allergic conditions can be very severe. Young children in particular may be plagued by eczema and food allergies. The latter may be life threatening. Peanut allergy is a particular case in point. Allergies to drugs and to latex can affect a person's health and quality of life. Allergic asthma even can reach the level of incapacitation or, rarely, death.

All of these disorders share a common mechanism; they reflect what has often been called type 2 immunity, named because the CD4 T cells that play a major role in many of these diseases are Th2 cells. Th2 cells produce a specific set of cytokines of which the index member is interleukin-4. IL-13, which is closely related to IL-4, is another critical product of these cells, as is a third cytokine, IL-5. The three cytokines act jointly to cause allergic inflammation. In the lung, allergic inflammation causes a buildup of mucus in the airways, an increased sensitivity of the airway to constrict in response to certain chemical mediators, and the influx of a population of inflammatory cells called *eosinophils*. Similar evidence of allergic inflammation can occur in the skin and in the intestinal tract.

IL-4, in addition to its mediation of allergic inflammation, is essential for the production of IgE, the form of antibody associated with allergic disease. IL-4 mediates the switching of B cells from cells in which the V_H genetic element is linked to $C\mu$ to cells in which V_H now lies in apposition to Cε and the H chain that these cells can produce is the εH chain that, when paired with an L chain, forms IgE.

Antibodies of the IgE class mediate many functions of allergy because their Fc region binds to specialized receptors (Fcε receptors) on two types of inflammatory cells, mast cells and basophils. When antibodies of the IgE class that are bound to Fcε receptors on mast cells and basophils interact with the antigens for which they are specific, an aggregation of the IgE-bound Fcε receptors occurs, triggering a biochemical reaction within the mast cell and the basophil that leads to the release of histamine and a series of related molecules often called *mediators*. These products cause constriction of airways and dilatation of blood vessels. Release of histamine and its congeners is responsible for many of the "mild" symptoms of allergy, but in some cases the immediate release of large amounts of histamine and other mediators can cause the individual to enter a state of shock, characterized by bronchial constriction, low blood pressure, hives, itching, and flushing. There is often severe swelling of the tongue or throat. This condition, *anaphylactic shock*, can be fatal. Anaphylactic shock is the constant worry of parents of children with severe food allergies, particularly to peanuts, and it is the reason why these children carry with them injectable adrenaline (in the form of EpiPens).

The incidence of allergies and asthma in children is rising dramatically throughout the world, most strikingly among some of the most advanced countries. It has been estimated that one in four children in New Zealand have asthma symptoms. It was anticipated that when populations of similar ethnic backgrounds living under different environmental conditions were compared for incidence of allergies and asthma, those who lived in the more polluted environment would have the higher incidence. However, when prevalence rates for asthma and allergic diseases were studied in the former West and East regions of the now unified Germany, prevalence was substantially higher in the West, despite lower degrees of pollution and presumably a healthier lifestyle. This result was mirrored in several other comparisons of populations of similar ethnicity living under very different circumstances. The finding that in countries in which populations benefit from low environmental pollution and, presumably, a cleaner environment, there is a greater, not a lower, incidence of allergic diseases and asthma, indicates a previously unrecognized cause of allergic diseases.

These observations led to the proposal of the *hygiene hypothesis*, which argues that in circumstances in which there is a higher incidence of childhood bacterial and or viral infections, the effect of such infections is to bias the individual's immune system to preferentially differentiate down the Th1 and/or Th17 pathways and to diminish the likelihood of the cells becoming Th2 cells. As the level of cleanliness rises and childhood infections become less prevalent, the argument is that this bias away from Th2 responses diminishes or is lost entirely and antigenic experiences are now more likely to elicit a Th2 response with an attendant allergic phenotype.

While this explanation has many attractive features, one must reserve a level of skepticism. Not only are immune conditions associated with type 2 immunity on the rise, there has also been a marked rise in the incidence of some autoimmune diseases that are based on Th1 or Th17 cells or perhaps CD8 cells. The incidence of type 1 diabetes is increasing in many parts of the world. Whether other autoimmune diseases are also increasing in prevalence is not clear. The diagnosis of these diseases may now be more certain and thus cases are being reported that would not have been discovered in the past. Nonetheless, we need to continue to examine the hygiene hypothesis and determine its true scope. What is clear is that allergic disorders are very common, particularly in the developed world, their prevalence is increasing, and they entail a serious burden of disease.

One question that invariably comes up is, what value does the type 2 immune response have? It surely did not evolve to cause diseases in the host. The T-cell component of the response plays an important role in resistance to helminthic infection. In infections with helminths, like hookworm or ascaris, a small intestinal roundworm, it is the type 2 response that is protective. In part, this is because IL-13, a Th2 product, plays a critical role in expulsion of the parasite, acting on gut epithelium and gut smooth muscle cells. Also, IL-5 mobilizes eosinophils that produce many antihelminthic substances.

The burden on human health of these helminthic infections, and thus the importance of Th2 responses, is very great. More than 200 million people are estimated to be infected with schistosomes. Schistosomaisis is one of the most devastating of the parasitic diseases, with an economic impact second only to malaria.

But what value does IgE serve? It acts in extremely low concentrations to mediate allergic inflammation. Does it have any positive role? It had generally been thought that it was a major mechanism through which helminthic parasites were eliminated. That may well be the case in humans, but thus far, in experimental animals, the role of IgE antibody in recovery from infection appears to be very limited. Of course, IgE must have a positive function or it would almost certainly have been lost in the course of evolution rather than being present in vertebrates for 160 million years.

Clearly, we need new ways to treat severe allergic inflammation or, even better, to anticipate who will develop these disorders, particularly severe eczema, major food allergies, and allergic asthma, and prevent them.

27

Interleukin-4 and Allergy

After Maureen Howard and I discovered interleukin-4 in 1982, Junichi Ohara and I uncovered the cell surface receptor through which IL-4 acts on its target cells and Graham Le Gros, Zami Ben-Sasson, and I devised methods to cause naïve CD4 T cells to develop into Th2 cells that produce IL-4 and its congeners on antigenic stimulation. This work turned out to be relevant to the study of type 2 immunity and IgE production and is having a major impact on the treatment of allergic inflammatory diseases.

Once Junichi Ohara, my postdoctoral fellow, had prepared IL-4 in chemically pure form, he and I collaborated with Ellen Vitetta in Dallas and with Bob Coffman in Palo Alto to show that IL-4 was critical to causing cells that originally expressed IgM on their membranes to switch to the expression of membrane IgG1 or IgE and eventually to become IgG1- or IgE-secreting cells.

How does the "switch event" occur? Ig class switching represents a second instance of gene rearrangement in which double strand breaks occur, allowing two genetic elements that had been far apart to be brought into apposition (figure 27.1). In IgE production, the assembled V_H genetic elements consist of contributions from V_H, D, and J_H gene segments. Between this assembled V_H element and the element encoding the constant region of IgM ($C\mu$) is a region designated the *switch region* for μ, Sμ. When cells are stimulated, physiologically in the germinal center or for experimental purposes in tissue culture, a double strand break occurs within Sμ and, in parallel, a double strand break also occurs in Sϵ, the switch region for ϵ, located just "upstream" of the constant region for IgE (Cϵ). IL-4 targets the

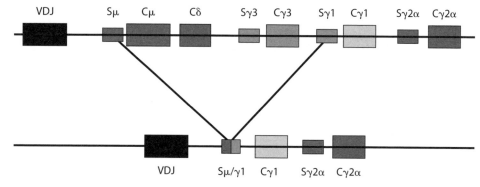

Figure 27.1. Mechanism of immunoglobulin class switching. Initially, IgM antibodies are produced, in which the μH chain consists of a VDJ H chain genetic element linked to the Cμ constant region. The DNA encoding the μ constant region (Cμ) is preceded by the Sμ switch region. In cells undergoing immunoglobulin class switching, a double strand break occurs within the Sμ switch region and in the switch region of one of the other C regions. In this illustration, the "upstream" portion of Sμ merges with the "downstream" portion of the γ1 switch region (Sγ1) to yield a rearranged Sμ/γ1 switch region. The VDJ variable region is now transcribed with Cγ1, yielding an IgG1 antibody.

Sε region to be the site of the "downstream" double strand break. The broken ends reseal in such a way that the upstream cut end from Sμ is annealed to the cut end from Sε, creating a new genetic element in which VDJ is followed by a hybrid Sμ/Sε switch region and then by Cε. When this region is transcribed (copied into mRNA) and then into protein, the V_H region that had originally been part of the IgM antibody is now part of an IgE antibody.

Switching thus represents a two-step procedure. One stimulant turns on the mechanism that leads to the double strand breaks. The second stimulant, IL-4, targets the downstream break to Sε and thus determines that switching will give rise to IgE.

With Ed Max, a talented molecular biologist in the FDA, Charles Chu and I designed a quantitative assay that allowed us to measure precisely the number of cells in which this rearrangement event had occurred. Our work with Bob Coffman had shown that if we stimulated B cells with LPS in tissue culture, which turned on the S region cleavage mechanism, and with IL-4, which targeted the Sε region for the rearrangement process, we obtained rearrangement and IgE production. While such tissue culture experiments are useful and allow one to work out the chemical mechanisms through which rearrangement occurs, they do not always reflect what occurs in the intact animal.

To determine whether IL-4 was essential for the production of IgE by experimental animals, we used a monoclonal anti-IL-4 antibody that Junichi Ohara had prepared. This monoclonal antibody, designated 11B11, binds to IL-4 in such a way as to block its activity. When Fred Finkelman, a former postdoc and longtime colleague, treated mice with a stimulant that induced a strong IgE response, we found that coadministration of 11B11 completely blocked IgE production. Others prepared mice from which the gene for IL-4 had been deleted. These mice were incapable of producing IgE. Thus, CD4 T cells that produce IL-4 are essential for the production of IgE, the class of antibody that is a major inducer of allergy.

In parallel with our study of IL-4-mediated immunoglobulin class switching to IgE, we also studied how IL-4 acts on its target cells. Junichi Ohara and I showed that IL-4 could bind very tightly to a cell surface molecule found on many cell types. This molecule was the IL-4 receptor. When IL-4 binds to its receptor, it results in a series of biochemical events in the cell that mediate IL-4's functions. We carried out a biochemical characterization of the IL-4 receptor and Achsah Keegan, Keats Nelms, and John Ryan analyzed the mechanisms through which the receptor mediates IL-4-determined functions. Regeneron Pharmaceuticals and its partner Sanofi have now developed a monoclonal antibody to the human IL-4 receptor, dupilumab, that has been quite effective in clinical trials for the treatment of moderate to severe allergic asthma and atopic dermatitis. This development proves that basic research on an interesting cytokine can lead to interventions that have the potential to better human health and shows the importance of IL-4 and its congener IL-13 in human allergic inflammatory diseases. But the time interval from discovery of the receptor to translation into a therapy for humans was far too long. Implementation of strategies to shorten the discovery–drug development period are essential.

Can the Immune System Control Cancer?

One of the greatest challenges of modern immunology is to understand the degree to which the immune system controls the growth of malignancies and whether specific immunity can be marshaled to prevent outgrowth of tumors or to treat existing tumors.

Immunosurveillance

The prevailing view is that the adaptive immune system evolved to provide protection against infectious agents—bacteria, viruses, parasites. An alternative idea is that the adaptive immune system developed in order to control the development of cancer cells. In complex, multicellular organisms such as vertebrates that contain trillions of cells, mutations will occur that lead some of these cells to develop unregulated growth, the first step toward malignancy. The recognition and elimination of such mutant cells by the immune system, it is argued, is essential for our survival. This process has been termed *immunosurveillance*. Even if adaptive immunity evolved initially to provide protection against infectious agents, it could easily have taken on immunosurveillance as a second important function.

Cancer cells undergo many mutations as they develop from their normal progenitors to the state of full malignancy. By virtue of such mutations, they contain many proteins that are different from the individual's native proteins. The immune system could certainly regard these mutant proteins as foreign and make an immune response against them. Responses to unique tumor antigens might eliminate cancer cells before they had developed into large tumors. Indeed, some suggest that the tumors that do develop are those that have escaped the control of the immune system because they are intrinsically of low immunogenicity, with those tumors of high immunogenicity having been eliminated.

However, an argument against the ubiquitous role of the immune system in preventing the development of cancer is that mice that have no adaptive immunity (mice in which genes essential for the development of the adaptive immune system have been deleted) do not develop many more malignancies than normal mice do, and the malignancies they do develop are often those of the immune system itself. This finding suggests that the development of malignancies may reflect the effect of the mutation on lymphocyte biology rather than a failure of immunosurveillance. But mice live for about two years, so the failure of immunoincompetent animals to develop cancers may simply mean that the process is time consuming. So, in this instance, the finding in mice may not be particularly valid for humans. Indeed, the success of checkpoint therapy, which I describe below, indicates that the immune system has a major role to play in controlling malignancy.

Immunity against Viruses Can Prevent Malignancy

What do we know about the role of the immune system in controlling cancer? There are some clear examples that immunity can limit the development of tumors. For example, vaccination against hepatitis B has had a remarkable effect in diminishing the incidence of liver cancer. This is particularly the case in East Asia, where liver cancer is quite common.

A study from Taiwan analyzed the incidence of liver cancer among children between the ages of six and fourteen.[1] For those born between 1975 and 1976, before the introduction of hepatitis B vaccine, the rate was 0.64 per 100,000 person years. Among those born between 1985 and 1986, after the vaccine was in general use, however, that rate had fallen to 0.1 per 100,000 person years, a reduction of 84 percent. The diminished incidence of liver cancer is truly remarkable. Based on this and other studies, it is likely that hepatitis B vaccination has prevented more cases of cancer than any other medical intervention apart from smoking cessation.

The recently introduced human papilloma virus vaccine is anticipated to cause a major reduction in cervical cancer, saving many lives, particularly among African women. Infection with certain types of human papilloma viruses induce the malignant process in cervical cells. Immunizing against the virus blocks the major pathway for the development of this malignancy.

Although these are two remarkable examples of the immune response's role in preventing induction of cancer, they do not deal with the actual elimination of malignant cells by the immune system but rather the more conventional action of the immune system to block viral infections. In both these cases, the virus is a major cause of the cancer; hepatitis B virus for liver cancers and human papilloma virus for cervical cancer. The immune system prevents cancer development not by killing the cancer cells but rather by preventing the virus infection, thus blocking the virus from inducing malignant transformation.

Let's turn to the question of whether the immune system can control cancer cells directly. Much early work was carried out by transplanting cancers from one mouse to another and determining whether the transplanted tumor cells could grow in the recipient. In these studies, care was not always taken to ensure that the donor and the recipient were fully "histocompatible," that is whether normal tissue from the tumor donor could be successfully transplanted to the recipient. Often, the transplanted tumor was rejected by the recipient not because the recipient had recognized antigens unique to the tumor (tumor antigens) but rather because the recipient had recognized antigens expressed on all tissue from the donor, including the tumor, that were foreign to the recipient. It was thought that transplantation was being used to study tumor immunity, but actually tumors were being used to study transplantation immunity.

However, there are clear examples of true tumor immunity. An elegant study carried out by Richmond Prehn and Joan Main working at the US Public Service Hospital in Seattle in the 1950s clearly demonstrated that some tumors did have specific antigens and that tumor-bearing mice could develop immunity to the tumors they carried.[2] Prehn and Main used a chemical that, when painted on the skin, was known to cause cancers to arise in mice. This chemical, methylcholanthrene, is a carcinogen. Prehn and Main produced twelve separate methylcholanthrene-induced sarcomas and transplanted each into individual mice of the same inbred strain. When the tumors reached a predetermined small size, they were removed surgically and, after a few days, the tumors were transplanted to new "naïve" mice, to the mouse from whom the tumor had been excised, and to other mice that had borne different tumors that had been excised. In ten of the twelve cases, the tumors grew in naïve mice, were rejected by the mice from whom the tumors had been taken, but grew when transplanted to mice that had borne a distinct tumor and from whom that tumor had been excised.

To be certain that this result was not due to an unrecognized difference in the mice (rather than in the tumors), normal skin from the tumor donor was also transplanted and, although the tumors were rejected, the normal skin was accepted, indicating that the mice were in fact histocompatible. The rejection of the tumors therefore implied that the tumor cells possessed an antigen that the normal skin did not.

This classic experiment proved that tumors could have specific tumor antigens and that, among the methylcholanthrene-induced sarcomas, each had a unique tumor antigen (or more likely, each had a unique set of tumor antigens). But the experiment gave us no information about whether naturally occurring tumors had tumor antigens. The methylcholanthrene-induced sarcomas were caused by the application of a powerful carcinogen to the skin and while some human tumors are no doubt caused by comparable carcinogens, most develop for other reasons.

Transplantation of experimental tumors continues to be used to gain insight into the regulation of tumor immunity and the nature of tumor antigens. In such experiments, tumors that have been derived from mice long ago and have been maintained either in tissue culture or by continuous transplantation into recipients are utilized. While these studies have been very valuable, revealing critical facts about how mice respond to tumors, there has always been the great worry that these tumors may not at all represent those that actually develop in humans.

One lesson from the study of these tumor transplantation models is that even in settings in which the tumor has an authentic tumor antigen, the tumor-bearing mouse may not reject the tumor. The tumor develops many defenses to protect itself against immune elimination. One strategy tumors use to protect themselves against killer T cells is to diminish the expression of major histocompatibility complex molecules and thus limit the display of their tumor antigens (see chapter 23). An evolved strategy of the host to deal with this problem is that natural killer cells recognize "missing self," that is, the absence or diminished amounts of class I MHC molecules on a tumor cell. When this recognition occurs, the NK cell is not inactivated by its inhibitory receptors and can attack the tumor.

Down-regulation of MHC molecules is only one of many mechanisms that tumors employ to protect themselves against immune attack. Other mechanisms through which tumor immunity is restrained include increased numbers of Tregs in the tumor tissue, diminished capacity of tumor-associated dendritic cells to act as potent antigen-presenting cells, the appearance of macrophages that are inhibitory to the immune response, the development of a metabolic environment that suppresses cells of the immune system, and the expression on the T cells of inhibitory receptors that diminish their function. These inhibitory receptors have become a target for drug development. The most carefully studied inhibitory receptor expressed by T cells is a molecule designated CTLA-4. Arlene Sharpe and her colleagues at Harvard Medical School showed that in the absence of CTLA-4, such as in genetically engineered mice in which the gene encoding CTLA-4 has been deleted, an uncontrolled generalized immune response occurs. These mice die by three to four weeks of age with their lymph nodes and spleens being massively enlarged and with immune destruction of their major organs.

The most detailed studies of CTLA-4 regulation of immunity have been carried out by Jim Allison. His work, together with the gene deletion work by Sharpe, clearly shows that inhibitory receptors such as CTLA-4 control immune responses, also implying that if activity of these receptors could be blocked, immune responses that had been inhibited might now be effective. Allison showed that monoclonal antibodies to mouse CTLA-4 would allow rejection of experimental tumors in mice. This finding encouraged him and his colleagues to push the idea that the development of monoclonal antibodies against human CTLA-4 could be effective in treatment of existing tumors by revealing a suppressed anti-tumor immunity.

A monoclonal antibody to human CTLA-4, ipilimumab, has been developed and shown in clinical trials to extend life in late-stage melanoma. Ipilimumab has been approved by the FDA and the European Union for the treatment of this cancer. In one trial, ipilimumab therapy extended life in late-stage melanoma from six months to ten months. While that may not seem to be a major effect, it is the first time any such effect had been achieved.

How does ipilimumab work? It is generally believed that when CTLA-4 is expressed on T cells, its engagement by ligands on antigen-presenting cells leads to an inhibition of the T cells' activation. The antibody, by blocking the interaction, frees the T cells of this inhibition. This implies that individuals who benefit from the treatment have T cells that are specific for the tumor antigen that have been inhibited in their function and are capable of controlling the tumor when freed of this inhibition.

However, there is an alternative view. CTLA-4 is expressed not only on conventional T cells; it is also found in large amounts on Tregs and, in some instances, CTLA-4 mediates the suppressive action of the Tregs. Thus, ipilimumab, by blocking CTLA-4, might prevent Tregs from suppressing the action of conventional T cells and thus reveal an ongoing immune response. Now that the drug is being widely used, it should be possible to determine which of the two alternatives is correct or, more likely, to what extent each contributes to the usefulness of the monoclonal antibody. This treatment has been termed *checkpoint therapy*. It relies on a normal function of the immune systems that, at a particular time in an immune response, makes a determination of whether a response is too exuberant and, if it is, restrains that response. Therapies that block this restraining activity are checkpoint therapies.

Another form of checkpoint therapy that researchers are investigating involves the molecule PD-1 (see chapter 19). The expression of PD-1 on killer T cells limits their activity, a physiologic response that prevented the development of immunopathology in those viral infections in which the infection did not result in cellular death. PD-1-mediated inhibition would limit both the killing of infected cells by killer T cells and the generalized inflammation resulting from excess production of IFNγ. Monoclonal antibodies to PD-1 have been developed and have proved effective in clinical trials in controlling a subset of lung cancers, renal cell cancer, and melanomas.

Blocking inhibitory receptors such as CTLA-4 and PD-1, while powerful and potentially very effective, has the disadvantage that it enhances all repressed immune responses and thus could have severe side effects arising from the development of autoimmune responses. A potentially better solution would be to find a way to regulate only the tumor-specific response itself, precisely targeting the defect in tumor-bearing patients. For such a strategy to work, we would need to know the nature of the tumor antigen and to find a way to selectively boost or derepress the anti-tumor immune cells. This would be most feasible if we could identify common tumor antigens expressed by all malignancies of a certain type. Indeed, the effort to develop anticancer vaccines is based on this concept.

Anti-tumor immunity is a very active area of study. Perhaps the first demonstration that shared tumor antigens existed came from the work of Thierry Boon and his colleagues in Brussels who showed that many human melanomas expressed an antigen they designated melanoma associated antigen-1 (MAGE-1). Efforts to boost immunity to MAGE-1 (or to more recently discovered homologs) might allow patients with melanomas that express the antigen to develop responses that would eliminate or shrink the tumor. Thus far, efforts to use MAGE-1-derived antigens in immunization have not met with clinical success, but the concept remains the "holy grail" of anti-tumor immunity.

Many other approaches to marshaling tumor-specific immunity are being studied. This is one of the most exciting, but also most frustrating, areas of modern immunology. That the immune system can be used to treat or prevent cancer was for many years only a hope, but the success of checkpoint therapy shows that it can be a reality. Yet it is clear we have far to go to realize the true promise of immune control of cancer.

New Parts for Old

Bone Marrow and Organ Transplantation

The idea of transplanting tissue to replace an injured or diseased organ is an ancient one. Using skin from one part of the body to help repair an injury to another part has a long history. Peter Medawar's wartime experiments worked out the rules governing the success or failure of such transplantation. His work made clear that skin grafts from a donor that was not a close major histocompatibility complex match to the recipient would inevitably be rejected and that a second graft from the same donor would be rejected more promptly. Transplantation was subject to the rules of immunology.

Blood Transfusion

The first great success of "transplantation," that is, of using foreign tissue to replace damaged tissues or host cells, was the transfusion of blood. Blood transfusion in the nineteenth century was far from a common practice, and on the rare occasions it was used, it was very much a hit or miss business, with some recipients benefitting and others suffering massive problems, often leading to death. The stage for modern blood transfusion as a safe and beneficial procedure was set by the discovery that human red blood cells were of different types and that the individual being transfused had preexisting immunity to blood types other than his or her own.

Karl Landsteiner, the individual who showed the vastness of the antigenic universe, discovered the ABO blood groups while working in Vienna in 1900. The ABO antigens are particular sugar molecules expressed on the surface of red blood cells. The ABO sugars are expressed on a major protein of the red cell as well as on a complex lipid. The relevant sugars are at the tip of a chain of other sugars. These "terminal" sugars are added to the sugar chain by the action of particular enzymes called glycosyl transferases. Individuals who are blood group A have a glycosyl transferase enzyme that adds the sugar N-acetylgalactosamine to the chain while individuals of group B have an enzyme that adds α-D-galactose. O group individuals lack either enzyme and do not add a terminal sugar.

Each of these enzymes is coded for by a gene; the ABO locus has three major alternative genetic forms (alleles); the A allele encodes the enzyme that adds N-acetylgalactosamine; the B allele encodes the enzyme that adds α-D-galactose; and the O allele encodes a nonfunctional enzyme. Each individual has two alleles at the ABO locus so individuals who are blood group A could have the genotype AA or AO; those who are blood group B are genotype BB or BO; blood group O individuals have the genotype OO; and those who are blood group AB have the genotype AB.

The A and B antigens are found on a variety of environmental substances so that A individuals will have become immunized to B and will have anti-B antibodies; B individuals will have anti-A antibodies; O individuals will have both anti-A and anti-B, and AB individuals will have neither. The development of these antibodies occurs early in life, and their presence is what makes an unmatched blood transfusion so dangerous.

Although we now recognize that there are many other antigenic differences on the red blood cells of different individuals, in general they are not of great importance for safe blood transfusion. However, there is one that deserves special attention. When Karl Landsteiner and his colleague Alexander Wiener immunized a rabbit with blood from a Rhesus macaque monkey, they obtained an antiserum that would bind to the red blood cells of some humans and not others. The genetics of the Rh (from Rhesus) system are more complicated than that of the ABO system and Rh-negative individuals do not spontaneously develop anti-Rh antibodies the way that anti-ABO antibodies develop.

Fetuses that have inherited Rh-positivity from their father but have an Rh-negative mother may develop hemolytic disease of the newborn or *erythroblastosis fetalis*. Women who are Rh-negative may produce anti-Rh antibodies if exposed to blood from an Rh-positive donor, or they may be sensitized as a result of having previously given birth to an Rh-positive infant. In subsequent pregnancies, the maternal anti-Rh antibodies cross the placenta, and if the fetus is Rh-positive, these antibodies can lead to destruction of the fetus's red blood cells with symptoms ranging from anemia to death.

Rh-negative women who are bearing an Rh-positive fetus for the first time can be treated with "Rh immune globulin," which itself does not destroy the fetus's red blood cells but prevents the mother from developing anti-Rh antibodies that would be destructive to the blood cells of Rh-positive fetuses in subsequent pregnancies. This treatment has had a great effect in lessening the number of cases of erythroblastosis fetalis.

While blood transfusion is obviously a triumph of transplantation, it does not provide a permanent replacement. Rather, blood cells have a limited lifespan in the recipient, as they had in the donor. The great accomplishments of the modern era of transplantation are the replacement of organs or bone marrow, leading to a permanent solution for individuals who require such replacement.

Kidney Transplantation

The first success of organ transplantation was the replacement of kidneys. Successful transplantation of kidneys and other organs presented two types of challenges: the technical problem of surgically implanting the organ in such a way that it would carry out its normal function and the immunological problem of preventing graft rejection because of histocompatibility differences between the donor and recipient. The initial success was to perfect the transplantation technique and the medical care of the transplant recipient. That was achieved by the expedient of carrying out a transplant between identical twins so that there was no problem of immunologically mediated graft rejection.

Joseph Murray, a surgeon at the Peter Bent Brigham Hospital (now Brigham and Women's Hospital) in Boston worked for two years to perfect the technique of kidney transplantation in dogs. With that background, he and his team were ready when Richard Herrick came to him with end-stage kidney disease. Richard's identical twin, Ronald, was prepared to donate a kidney. On December 23, 1954, the transplant was carried out. The operation was a success and Richard Herrick survived for eight years after the surgery.[1]

Once it was demonstrated that kidney transplantation was technically feasible, the great challenge was how to do it successfully for individuals who did not have an identical twin. Two parallel approaches were important—finding ways to limit the recipient's immune response and finding donors as close as possible to the recipient in histocompatibility type. The latter provided a great incentive to study the human histocompatibility antigens in detail and to find quick and reliable typing methods. There are three major linked genetic loci encoding human class I MHC molecules, HLA-A, B, and C, and three encoding human class II MHC molecules, HLA-DP, DQ, and DR. The number of variants at each locus is very large, so finding good matches is often very difficult.

In the United States, approximately one-third of all transplants are from living donors. Often a sibling is willing to donate. In one case in four, a sib can be expected to be a complete match, but this means that 75 percent of the time any individual sib is not. In order to find good matches for individuals with willing but unmatched donors, what has evolved is a process called *kidney chains*. Basically, by HLA typing and using sophisticated computer programs, a potential donor for a recipient who has an unmatched but willing donor is identified; a recipient for that individual's unmatched potential donor is then found and the process goes on. In 2012, there was a kidney chain involving thirty donors, thirty recipients, and seventeen hospitals.[2]

The other great advance that has made kidney and other organ grafts so successful has been the use of drugs that suppress the immune system. It was to this that Joseph Murray directed his attention after his success in grafting a kidney from one twin to another. Even in well-matched donor-recipient pairs, there are minor histocompatibility differences, and in many cases matching is not complete. Thus, immunosuppression continues to be essential for maintenance of a kidney graft.

Murray working with a young British surgeon, Ray Calne, collaborated with George Hitchings and Gertrude Elion at the Burroughs Wellcome & Co. pharmaceutical firm. Hitchings and Elion were developing immunosuppressive drugs, one of which was azathioprine, which continues to be used today. Azathioprine proved very useful in suppressing recipients' immune responses so they would accept and retain kidneys that were not perfectly matched. This launched kidney transplantation as a feasible treatment for many individuals with end-stage kidney disease.

Each of the contributors to this success has been honored in many ways. Murray received the 1990 Nobel Prize in Physiology or Medicine, which he shared with E. Donnal Thomas, the pioneer in bone marrow transplantation. Hitchings and Elion received the 1988 Nobel Prize for their drug development work. Roy Calne (later Sir Roy Calne) shared the 2012 Lasker Clinical Prize with Thomas Starzl (on whom, more below). And the HLA typing accomplishments were not ignored. Jean Dausset received the 1980 Nobel Prize for his work on HLA antigens, shared with my mentor Baruj Benacerraf and George Snell, who had pioneered the study of the mouse major histocompatibility complex.

The most important immunosuppressive drugs proved to be cyclosporine A (CsA) and its congener FK-506 or tacrolimus. These drugs block the action of the enzyme *calcineurin*. Calcineurin removes phosphates from a transcription factor called NFAT. The removal of phosphates from NFAT allows it to enter the nucleus, where it plays a critical role in the production of cytokines, such as interleukin-2, that are important for immune responses. CsA and tacrolimus, by blocking the action of calcineurin, prevent the production of IL-2 and related cytokines and thus inhibit immune responses. Even CsA needs to be supplemented with other immunosuppressive agents. Consequently, graft recipients may suffer from the side effects of the immunosuppressive drugs and are at risk of infection because of their chronic immunosuppression.

Kidney transplantation is a major success story. The greatest difficulty is the shortage of kidneys. In the United States, approximately 98,000 individuals are on the waiting list for a kidney.[3] More than 16,000 kidney transplants were done in 2012. Since the majority of kidneys come from deceased individuals, particularly those who die in accidents, a greater willingness of the population at large to be potential organ donors could help to deal with this long backlog.

Liver and Bone Marrow Transplantation

Transplantation of many other organs is now possible. Among the types of transplants that are done are heart, lung, heart-lung combinations, pancreas, intestine, stomach, corneas, islets of Langerhans, and face. More than 6,000 liver transplants are performed each year.

The technical problems in liver transplantation were much more formidable than for kidneys. Through a stepwise process, Thomas Starzl in the United States and Roy Calne in the UK developed the modern highly successful surgical techniques that make liver transplantation almost routine. But it was the introduction of highly effective immunosuppressive drugs that has made survival of transplanted livers possible. Calne and

Starzl led the way to the use of CsA so that today liver transplantation is a safe, effective, and lifesaving treatment.

Another procedure that has seen significant success is bone marrow transplantation. Scientists had long known that patients with leukemia could clearly benefit from replacing all their blood-forming cells with cells from a normal individual. This would eliminate all the leukemic cells and replace them with blood-forming cells from a normal donor. The challenge was to find a way to destroy the leukemic cells as completely as possible and then, since that would almost certainly destroy all the normal blood-forming cells, to safely reconstitute the blood-forming system. Some of the earliest efforts to carry out bone marrow transplantation were done not in patients with leukemia but in individuals who had been exposed to large doses of radiation.

E. Donnal Thomas and his colleagues at the Fred Hutchison Cancer Center in Seattle were among the pioneers in the effort to develop successful bone marrow transplantation. As early as 1959, when Thomas was still at the Mary Imogene Bassett Hospital in Cooperstown, New York, he carried out bone marrow transplants in individuals with leukemia in which the donor and recipient were identical twins. The recipient was first exposed to high doses of irradiation in an attempt to eliminate all the leukemic cells and to make "space" for the transplanted bone marrow. In two cases, successful reconstitution of the hematopoietic cells and remission of the leukemia was achieved, but, unfortunately, the patients' leukemia returned after a few months. These experiments proved that bone marrow could be transplanted and that, at least in the short term, this might be an approach to treat leukemia.

In kidney and liver grafts some incompatibility can be tolerated with the availability of modern immunosuppressive drugs. But in bone marrow transplantation, HLA matching is of great importance. The progress in the knowledge of the HLA system and improved methods of typing made it possible for Thomas and his colleagues to return to the field of transplantation in the late 1960s with related but non-twin donors.

In the interim, Dr. Robert Good, at the University of Minnesota, carried out a successful transplant from a matched sibling into an infant with a severe combined immunodeficiency disease. This was an easier problem than transplantation for the treatment of leukemia because the preparation of the patient is less rigorous. It wasn't essential that the patient's bone marrow be completely ablated since there was no leukemia to destroy, and since the patient had an immune defect, he could not reject the transferred cells. The transplant was a success, and the child had a long and healthy life. Indeed, at Robert Good's eightieth birthday celebration in 2002, the transplant recipient and his mother were honored guests.

Thomas returned to bone marrow transplantation in patients with leukemia using bone marrow from matched sibling donors in 1969, and by 1975 he had carried out seventy transplants in patients with acute leukemia and thirty-seven in patients with aplastic anemia, a disease in which there is bone marrow failure. His results in aplastic anemia were encouraging; half the recipients had survived for three years. The results in acute leukemia were less positive, but some of the recipients had survived for four years. While some succumbed to a recurrence of their leukemia, many fell victim to a reaction of the lymphocytes from the bone marrow graft against the tissues of the recipient, a condition known as *graft-versus-host disease*, which is a major problem in bone marrow transplantation between nonidentical donor-recipient pairs.

With the passage of time, better preparation of the patients, better treatment of their leukemia, and better immunosuppression to prevent or manage graft-versus-host disease has markedly improved the results in bone marrow transplantation for leukemia. Indeed, bone marrow is no longer the only source of cells that could be transplanted to restore the blood-forming system of an individual. The cells that mediate this function, *hematopoietic stem cells* (HSCs) (*hematopoiesis* is the formation of blood cellular components), can be mobilized into the blood by certain treatments, sparing the donor of the somewhat painful procedure of harvesting bone marrow. Another source of HSCs is umbilical cord blood. Today, the term *hematopoietic cell transplant* is probably more appropriate than bone marrow transplant. By whatever name one prefers, this is now a lifesaving therapy. In 2011, approximately 7,500 hematopoietic cell transplants were performed in the United States in which the donor and recipient were not identical twins.

Hematopoietic cell transplantation is used for the various leukemic conditions, for primary immunodeficiency diseases, and for diseases in which key enzymes essential for normal metabolism are absent or nonfunctional. Indeed, the list of conditions in which hematopoietic cell transplant can be considered as a therapy continues to grow.

30

Julien

Nature's first green is gold,
Her hardest hue to hold.
Her early leafs a flower;
But only so an hour.

—Robert Frost, "Nothing Gold Can Stay"

This chapter deals with a painful episode in our family's history, but I relate it since it gives a human scale to the story of hematopoietic stem cell transplantation, illustrating both its hope and, tragically, its failures.

My son Matthew and his wife, Naomi Mezey, today have a son, Jake, and a daughter, Lucy. Jake was born in 1999, and in 2001, his brother, Julien, made his appearance. Lucy came later, in 2005, after the events I am about to recount had transpired. Julien was an apparently healthy infant and soon revealed himself to be a feisty, adventurous little boy, a joy to all around him (see figure 30.1).

From his earliest pediatrician visits, all seemed well, with the exception that his platelet counts were quite low. Platelets are small cells (actually fragments of large cells, megakaryocytes) that play an important role in blood clotting. Julien's pediatrician was not too concerned about his thrombocytopenia (*thrombocyte* is a synonym for platelet, and *penia* indicates diminished cell numbers). But with successive visits, Julien's platelet counts fell rather than correcting. On one occasion, I was visiting Duke University School of Medicine, where Michael Frank, a close friend, was chairman of the Department of Pediatrics. Mike suggested that I discuss Julien's platelet issues with the head of the Division of Pediatric Hematol-

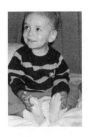

Figure 30.1. Julien Mezey, our beloved JJ. (Courtesy of Matthew Paul and Naomi Mezey)

ogy. The hematologist was optimistic; many infants have low platelet counts, which they usually tolerate quite well, and which correct themselves as the infants get older.

Unfortunately, Julien's problem did not correct itself, and by the time he was a year and a half old, it became clear that there was a much more sinister explanation for the platelet deficiency. Blast cells appeared in his blood, a sign of a leukemia that particularly affects the cells that give rise to platelets, a type of acute myeloid leukemia (AML) that is particularly difficult to treat.

Matt and Naomi consulted several pediatricians and were referred to Children's Hospital in Washington where the diagnosis of AML of the M7 type (acute megakaryoblastic leukemia) was confirmed. Julien was admitted to the hospital and was treated with a combination of chemo-therapeutic agents in an effort to place him in remission. The goal was to achieve remission and, since there was a high risk of relapse in this disease, to follow this with a hematopoietic stem cell transplant.

This began a long period of hospitalization for Julien during which one of his parents was always with him. The treatment that began at Children's and continued later took its toll on this previously carefree and joyful little boy. But the nurses at Children's Hospital were outstanding. The women (almost all of Julien's nurses were women) who cared for him and for other children with leukemia are remarkable in their caring attitude, their devotion to their patients, and their ability to be cheerful in the face of potential tragedy.

While Julien tolerated the chemotherapy reasonably well, there was some uncertainty as to how effective it was. The physicians at Children's were of the opinion that Julien had entered remission, but when we consulted those who were to do the hematopoietic stem cell transplant, their view was that the remission was incomplete at best.

The problem was what to do next. It was clear that a transplant was needed, but there were options as to the type of transplant and where to do it. An immediate concern was, if a bone marrow transplant were to be done, could we find a matched donor?

Jake was typed in the hope that he would prove to be a match. As I mentioned earlier, there are three major class I HLA antigens (HLA-A, B, and C) and three major class II HLA antigens (HLA-DP, DQ, and DR). Each antigen is coded for by an HLA gene; since the genes are located close to one another, they are generally inherited as a unit. Each brother would have received one copy of this HLA unit from Matt and one copy from Naomi. Thus, there was a 25 percent chance that both brothers would be matched at the six genetic loci. Unfortunately, Jake and Julien shared one gene set but differed at the second.

Since Jake was not a suitable donor, the choice was to find a match by searching various databases. While Matt and Naomi were considering their options, the search process began. At that time, the search was an automated one through the National Marrow Donor Program, now replaced by "Be the Match" online registry.

While Julien was hospitalized at Children's Hospital, a drive was organized to sign up as many potential bone marrow donors as possible to expand the pool of individuals in the National Marrow Donor Program. The Red Cross provided the infrastructure for the drive, which was held at the Georgetown University Law School, where Naomi is a professor. We had a terrific turnout of people from the law school, from Matt's law firm at the time, Patton Boggs, from Marilyn's colleagues at the National Archives, from mine at NIH, and from friends throughout the Washington area. A blood sample was taken from each for typing purposes.

Events such as this expand the donor pool so that the chances of finding a match are improved for all who need a transplant. Of course, people are motivated to help because of a connection to an affected child or adult, but by participating they are potentially benefiting all by expanding the number of individuals in the donor program.

The matching program also accesses another set of banks of cells available for transplantation: umbilical cord blood units, blood taken from the umbilical cord after birth. Such blood is a good source of stem cells, and since the lymphocytes in the cord blood are relatively immature, these cells are somewhat less likely to cause graft-versus-host disease. For that reason, transplants can be done with umbilical cord blood with a slightly less good match than that required for a bone marrow transplant.

One disadvantage of umbilical cord blood is that the sample usually contains fewer stem cells than bone marrow taken from an adult does. However, if the recipient is a child, a typical unit of umbilical cord blood may have sufficient stem cells for a successful transplant.

There are many excellent hematopoietic stem cell transplant programs, including several that specialize in children. We spoke to Rich O'Reilly at Memorial Hospital in New York City and to David Nathan at Boston Children's Hospital, both of whom were very helpful and encouraged Matt and Naomi to consider having the transplant done at their hospitals. In the end, the choice came down to two truly outstanding programs for pediatric hematopoietic stem cell transplantation, the University of Minnesota and Duke. Matt and Naomi chose Duke because of its excellent program in transplanting children and its concentration on umbilical cord blood transplants, and because of the dynamic and caring leader of its program, Dr. Joanne Kurtzberg.

One advantage of the umbilical cord blood transplant was how quickly it could be carried out, because the units were already "banked" in frozen form. This was a particular concern as Joanne Kurtzberg, on reviewing Julien's blood smears, was not convinced that he had entered a complete remission.

So, in the summer of 2003, Matt and Naomi brought Julien and Jake to Durham for what would be six months, first staying with Ruth and Michael Frank and then renting a small house close to Duke Hospital. Julien was immediately admitted, and the process of preparing him for the transplant began. This involved the use of high doses of drugs that would destroy Julien's own blood-forming cells and the leukemia cells. The doses used were higher than in the initial chemotherapy since it was not necessary to be concerned about sparing normal cells. Those cells would be replaced by the donor's cells. Matt or Naomi continued to be present at Julien's bedside around the clock, although occasionally Marilyn or I would spell them for a few hours.

A cord blood unit with a fairly good match was available at Duke and so, once Julien's preparation was completed, we all held our breath while the unit was infused. Then, it was a matter of waiting. The first hurdle was to find evidence that the transplanted stem cells had engrafted. Until engraftment occurred, Julien would be effectively without any immune system or any blood cells at all. He needed both blood and platelet transfusions and even transfusions of neutrophils.

Since umbilical cord blood has fewer stem cells than the typical amount available from bone marrow, engraftment takes longer. In Julien's case, it took a particularly long time but we celebrated when his blood counts started to rise. Of course, he required potent immunosuppressive drugs to prevent the grafted cells from reacting against his tissues in the dreaded graft-versus-host disease.

But we were gratified that his counts continued to rise, and there was no evidence of leukemic cells. The staff at Duke was truly amazing, from leader Joanne Kurtzberg to every member of the staff. Joanne was a bundle of energy, completely devoted to her many patients.

After a few months in the hospital, Julien was allowed to go home to the rented house in Durham, wearing a face mask whenever he was around other than family members. In December, Julien celebrated his second birthday in Durham with a great cake and family, especially big brother Jake, then four and a half, in attendance. Six months after their arrival at Duke, in January 2004, Dr. Kurtzberg deemed that Julien could return to the Mezey-Paul home in Washington, DC.

Arrangements were made with the leukemia group at Georgetown University Hospital to be available for Julien's care, and Dr. Kurtzberg continued to be deeply involved. All seemed to go well, but in late February, Julien developed a fever and was admitted to Georgetown University Hospital. Crushing news came from the physicians there. Blast cells had returned to his blood, signifying a relapse of his leukemia.

Joanne Kurtzberg and the doctors at Georgetown thought the best course was to take Julien off his immunosuppressive drugs, hoping that the donor T cells would display a "graft-versus-leukemia" effect and eliminate the malignant cells. Whether this may have worked wasn't clear, but what was clear is how devastating graft-versus-host reactions can be when the drugs are removed. Julien developed all the classical signs of the attack of the donor T cells against his tissue, despite what had been a good match. The most obvious problem was severe skin rash, but the T cells attacked virtually every organ and, as far as could be told, the leukemia was back in full force, also taking a terrific toll on this little boy.

We watched helplessly as he experienced the ravages of the two diseases and finally, the worst. Julien died on March 29, 2004.

He was buried in the Academy Cemetery in Clovis, California, a cemetery that members of Naomi's family had helped to found in the 1800s. His grave is under a spreading tree with a view of the foothills of the Sierras. In his memory, the Association for the Study of Law, Culture, and the Humanities, of which Naomi was an important member, established the Julien Mezey Dissertation Award.[1]

While we have come a long way in the effort to treat leukemia and all cancers by using the tools of immunity and of transplantation, much remains to be done. Julien's short life illustrates the hope and the reality of hematopoietic stem cell transplantation for the treatment of leukemia.

Conclusion

The Future of Immunology

Predicting the future is a perilous enterprise. Even the predictions of eminent scientists have proven dismal failures.

First, however, a prediction that wasn't a failure. In an address to the Second International Congress of Mathematicians in Paris in 1900,[1] David Hilbert, one of the greatest mathematicians of the nineteenth and twentieth centuries, proposed twenty-three problems that laid out much of the program of mathematics for the coming century. This farseeing "prediction" was vastly influential in shaping the development of mathematics over more than a hundred years.

By contrast, two contemporaries of Hilbert's, both distinguished figures, made predictions that are rather embarrassing to read now. One, Albert Michelson, was the first American to win the Nobel Prize in Physics. In 1894, Michelson said, "The more important fundamental laws and facts of physical science have all been discovered, and these are so firmly established that the possibility of their ever being supplanted in consequence of new discoveries is exceedingly remote . . . our future discoveries must be looked for in the sixth place of decimals."[2] And around 1900, Lord Kelvin, one of the great physicists of the nineteenth century and a president of the Royal Society, was quoted as saying, "There is nothing new to be discovered in physics now. All that remains is more and more precise measurement."[3] Just a few years later, relativity and quantum theory shook the foundations of physics and led to completely new worldviews.

Recognizing the danger, I want to venture a few comments about the future of immunology. In terms of accomplishment, I look to the development of new families of vaccines that will overcome the great scourges of humankind, including AIDS, tuberculosis, and malaria. Similarly, a deeper knowledge of the mechanistic basis of the autoimmune diseases should lead us to better and better interventions and, best of all, to ways to predict and prevent these diseases. Whether immunology can "cure" cancer is beyond my predictive power, but I am encouraged by the success of checkpoint therapies and believe that strategies to overcome many of the inhibitory mechanisms that tumors have developed to restrain the immune response can make a major difference in the efficacy of immunologically based cancer treatment.

Furthermore, understanding the mechanisms through which the microbial contents of our intestines (the intestinal microbiome) control many aspects of immunity and inflammation may provide the means to improve the function of many organ systems. We have seen how a disordered microbiome led to fatty liver disease in experimental animals and thus potentially to metabolic syndrome and type 2 diabetes (chapter 22). I am confident we will learn what components of the microbiome are key to promoting health and which components are pro-inflammatory. Then we will be able to regulate the bacteria in our gastrointestinal tract to optimize health by controlling inflammation on a systemwide basis.

But perhaps more important than the particular discoveries that will be made are the fundamental changes in the strategies that immunologists, and indeed all biomedical scientists, will use to tackle important problems, particularly those related to human disease. I believe we are now at a tipping point in biomedical science. The range of new technologies that have been introduced over the last several years and those that we can expect shortly will fundamentally alter how many of us do science. They will allow us to address problems that today are clearly beyond our reach. To a degree, some of these changes are already finding their way into the biomedical science enterprise, so perhaps it is unfair to class them as predictions. Nonetheless, I believe that implementing these approaches will have an enormous impact on the future of immunology.

Virtually all the breakthroughs I describe in this book had their roots in basic discoveries that came from animal experiments. Indeed, the majority of the newly introduced drugs that are proving so successful in controlling immune and inflammatory diseases and cancer can be traced directly to research in experimental animals, in particular inbred mice. Sadly, the time from discovery to application to humans has been painfully long. It was 1987 when Junichi Ohara and I first identified and characterized the cell surface receptor through which the cytokine interleukin-4 signals (chapter 18).[4] In 2013, twenty-six years later, clinical trials of dupilumab, a monoclonal anti-human-IL-4 receptor antibody, revealed encouraging results in the treatment of atopic dermatitis and in moderate-to-severe allergic asthma.[5] And, if these trials are followed by successful phase III trials, as I very much hope they will be, the delay until the monoclonal antibody is available as a human therapeutic will be even longer. How can we shorten the time from discovery to application and, equally importantly, concentrate our development efforts on areas that strongly affect human physiology and human disease?

Using Heritable Human Disorders to Understand the Molecular Basis of Disease

While the basic principles of immune function are similar in humans and mice, the details of human and mouse immunology are, of course, not the same. Until recently, we have accepted that this problem existed and have rather painfully moved through a process of discovery in the mouse, creation of in vivo models in mice, analysis of the cellular and biochemical pathways involved, determination of whether similar effects are seen in the in vitro analysis of human cells, and finally investigation of whether these mechanisms are important in human physiology. Often, the key test is a clinical trial to examine the effects of a drug that targets the putative pathway. All too often, a drug whose usefulness was anticipated based on animal studies fails in human trials.

I would be the last to argue against the use of experimental animal systems to discover the basic principles underlying human immunity and disease abnormalities. Studies of the inbred mouse will continue to yield key insights into the biology of immunity and reveal new principles underlying immune functioning. Yet I think that we need to reorganize a significant fraction of our efforts and to begin with human analysis and then to study in detail the findings proven to be important in the human, in experimental animal systems. This is more possible now than it would have been even a few years ago because of technological advances.

One of the surest ways to discover a function important in humans is to observe the consequences of the failure of that function. While we have always known of individuals and families in which there were severe, heritable immunological abnormalities, the cause of these abnormalities could be determined in only a limited number of cases. But that has changed. Modern techniques of genome sequencing and measurement of gene expression now make it possible in the majority of cases to rapidly determine the genetic basis of heritable disorders of immunity (and indeed of all human functions).

One of the great virtues of studying human immune diseases is that when a failure of some process leads to a severe abnormality, the individual in whom the failure occurs will almost always be brought to a physician's attention. If these abnormalities are familial or if they affect a young child, there is a reasonable likelihood they may be caused by a mutation in a single gene.

The discovery of a mutant gene that leads to a major immunologic abnormality pinpoints a biochemical "pathway" that is critical to immune function in humans. Modern techniques of gene sequencing now allow whole genomes to be sequenced at relatively low cost, and advances in bioinformatics allow the rapid identification of the mutant gene. This information provides us with the molecular basis for the particular disease. As the number of identified disease-causing mutations grows, we will amass a database of human pathways that are critical for normal function of a wide range of physiologic systems.

Analyzing how these prevalidated biochemical pathways actually function, and how they intersect with one another, still will require working in animal models, but here too, the pace should speed up. Newer techniques are available for preparing genetically manipulated mice in which given pathways are blocked as a result of deleting or mutating key genes. These animal models allow a thorough exploration of the impact of the pathway under a variety of conditions and help determine how cells bearing particular mutations actually function within the animal.

I would estimate the time from a discovery that a particular gene contributes to a human disorder to understanding the mechanism underlying the process could be shortened to a few years so that the process of looking for compounds that can block molecular targets could start much sooner, readying drugs to test in the clinic in a relatively short time rather than in a decades-long interval. Thus, the molecular basis of human genetic disease would be prevalidated. The exploitation of this knowledge in experimental animal systems and in human cells will help us not only to plan treatments of the rare individuals who have these genetically determined disorders but also, more importantly, to establish the centrality of the involved pathway in its function in common diseases within the general population.

Thus, the path of discovery will be altered. It will flow from the recognition of a heritable human disease, to discovery of the genetic mutation underlying the disease, to deep analysis of the biochemical pathway, to the analysis of abnormalities in genetically manipulated mice, to the application of this detailed knowledge to common human immunologic diseases. This course of action has the advantage that we will not be distracted by those detailed mechanisms that pertain in an experimental animal but not in a human; thus, we can keep our path of discovery concentrated in areas that we are certain are relevant for human disease. New technologies should speed the entire process.

As always, there is an important caveat. While I regard this new process as the royal road to studying the basis of human disease, and thus to the development of effective drugs, there must always been a major carving out of resources and programs that allow the discovery of the entirely unanticipated mechanisms, often only approachable in animal systems. The reorganization of our efforts cannot crowd out this central proven pathway to new knowledge.

Using Big Data to Discover Causal Effects and Assess Human Variability

A second revolutionary approach is to combine our increasingly powerful analytical tools with modern computational approaches to seek out associations between sets of measurements of patient characteristics and outcomes in various treatments or prevention strategies. For example, performing whole genome sequencing for a sufficiently large number of individuals, profiling patterns of expressed genes in these individuals, and linking these with a database of their detailed health records should allow a determination of whether allelic forms (rare or common) at given genetic loci or epigenetic changes at such loci are associated with heightened (or diminished) susceptibility to particular diseases, and with responsiveness to particular treatments. Such great progress is being made in genome and RNA sequencing that it will soon be feasible to have complete genomic sequences on virtually every individual, as well as measurements of his or her patterns of gene expression. These advances will be coupled with advances in data analysis so that computational methods to find associations between genes and disease will become more and more reliable.

For example, collecting both genomic and gene expression information from a large number of individuals who receive a given vaccine or who become infected with a particular pathogen and determining their responses can lead to critical insights. Computational biologists can seek to identify quantitative changes in sets of expressed molecules that correlate to a very high degree with a good or bad outcome. Take the recent effort to understand why the yellow fever vaccine is so good. The currently used vaccine (17D), an attenuated live virus, was first tested in 1938. It has proven to be remarkably effective, with over 400 million doses administered. But until 2014 we knew very little about why 17D is such a successful vaccine.

Bali Pulendran and his colleagues at the Emory Vaccine Center in Atlanta compared the immune response of a large number of people vaccinated with 17D with gene expression profiles in those individuals.[6] They identified a gene that showed a high degree of correlation between the degree of its induction and the strength of the immune response to the vaccine. When they studied this gene, designated GCN2, the team found that it programmed dendritic cells for enhanced antigen-presenting function through a cellular mechanism called *autophagy*. This was an unanticipated molecular pathway for enhancing the antigen-presenting function of dendritic cells, and it not only explained why 17D was so good but also pointed the way to improve other vaccines. It even may have wider significance for enhancing immune responses in general. Thus, large data sets of this type analyzed with powerful computational tools provide a second approach to discovery of critical pathways associated with certain outcomes in humans.

Big data (also known as data science) also gives us a window on human variability and should allow us to distinguish those patients for whom a therapy is likely to be effective from those in whom it would very likely fail. Big data can provide patient stratification for therapy and for understanding the variable pathways that lead to disease in a population as diverse as humans.

This prescription for new ways to do science has to be applied carefully. The most certain thing about the future is that it will produce the unexpected, and while we must position ourselves to take advantage of new and powerful technologies, we must keep a solid place for the kinds of insights that may only come through creative flashes, often based on unusual behaviors observed in experimental animal systems.

Epilogue

While we have learned much about the mechanisms that underlie the remarkable human immune system, and while the accomplishments of immunologists are many and of great importance, our knowledge is far from complete. Preventives, cures, and treatments for many diseases with immunologic components still elude us.

The path that brought us to what we know now depended on fundamental research and the subsequent application of that research to illuminating the human immune system and how it behaves in disease. The great success of this effort has been due in very large part to the investment made, particularly by the people of the United States and other nations, to support the biomedical research enterprise. This investment has brought virtually all the pathbreaking insights described in these pages, and it has supported my own research effort and that of my colleagues since 1961 when I began work in Alan Cohen's laboratory at the Boston University Medical Center.

Funds to support research in the biomedical sciences in the United States are mainly provided by the National Institutes of Health. The majority are distributed in the form of research grants to scientists working at universities, medical schools, research institutes, and hospitals across the country whose proposals have successfully weathered a rigorous peer review.

Approximately 10 percent of federal funds are spent in the intramural research program on the campus of the National Institutes of Health, in Bethesda, Maryland, where I have worked throughout my entire career as an independent scientist. Here, too, a rigorous review is carried out to ensure that the very best research is supported.

But we now face a dilemma. The progress in contemporary science has been truly remarkable. A whole new tool kit has become available, allowing types of experiments to be done and insights to be obtained that were simply beyond our reach even a few years ago. The exploitation of these new approaches, building on the knowledge we have already obtained, promises to yield explanations for the many still vexing problems, to strike at the root causes of many of the autoimmune and inflammatory diseases, and to lead us to strategies to prevent, cure, or treat these diseases, as well to develop new therapies for cancer.

But, sadly, resources are shrinking at the very time that opportunities are expanding. The American people, acting through the Congress and the administration, had assigned a high value to medical research. Indeed, in the period between 1950 and 2003, the NIH appropriation increased from $500 million to $27.2 billion, representing an approximately 8 percent annual growth rate. This increase from a very modest start has allowed US biomedical science to lead the world. One impressive but imperfect statistic is that in this same period, 87 of the 148 scientists who won a Nobel Prize in Physiology or Medicine were US citizens.

By contrast, since 2004, the NIH budget has been essentially stagnant, rising from $28 billion in 2004 only to $30.9 billion in 2012, a yearly increase of 1 percent, well below the rate of inflation of the cost of biomedical research. Indeed, between 2010 and 2012, the budget fell each year. Even the most effective scientists have found getting grants to support their research increasingly difficult. The success rate (the number of grant applications funded divided by the number submitted) has dropped from 30 percent in 2003 to 19 percent in 2012. Effectively that means that many talented individuals, particularly younger scientists, will fail to obtain research support and may leave science, cutting off a future generation of leaders in our field. Unless we take steps to ensure a reasonable investment in medical research, particularly in basic research, the rate of scientific progress will slow. While other countries may pick up some of the slack, the US research establishment is the world's largest and most sophisticated. If it stumbles, the implications for progress for all are dire.

But I don't wish to end on a sour note. Science has proven over and over that it is the surest way to human progress. The history of this progress, in virtually every discipline, is a fascinating one. An understanding of the process, with its missteps and great successes, provides us with the tools to evaluate the claims of tomorrow, and it should allow each of us, as citizens, to play our role in making the critical choices that will prepare us for the future.

Acknowledgments

I offer my thanks to the many individuals who took the time to read all or part of the book and who offered useful suggestions. They include Maria Freire of the Foundation for the National Institutes of Health; Zvi Grossman of the Sackler School of Medicine at Tel Aviv University; Siamon Gordon of Oxford University; and Harold Varmus of the National Cancer Institute. I particularly wish to thank my son, Jonathan Carmel, for his suggestions to improve the book and make it more accessible to the general reader and my wife, Marilyn Paul, for her continued support and her incisive comments. I thank my son and daughter-in-law, Matthew Paul and Naomi Mezey, for their permission to discuss their son Julien Mezey's illness, transplant, and all that followed.

Many individuals provided materials used in the illustrations, which I have acknowledged in the figure legends. I particularly thank Dr. Stephane Caucheteux for his gift of the stamp honoring Pasteur's introduction of the rabies vaccine and Dr. Georg Stingl for his gift of the Austrian note honoring Karl Landsteiner.

The editorial staff at Johns Hopkins University Press provided outstanding advice and counsel. I wish particularly to acknowledge the help of Jacqueline Wehmueller, Kelley Squazzo, Robin Coleman, and Isla Hamilton-Short. I also thank Glenn Perkins for his outstanding copyediting and for numerous excellent suggestions to improve my explanation of often complex issues.

Notes

Chapter 1. Defense and Danger

1. Edward Jenner, *The Three Original Publications on Vaccination against Smallpox*, Harvard Classics ed. (New York: P. F. Collier & Son, 1909–14; Bartleby.com, 2001, www.bartleby.com/38/4/).

2. For a discussion of variolation, see the National Library of Medicine at www.nlm.nih.gov/exhibition/smallpox/sp_variolation.html.

3. Abigail Adams took four of her children to Boston to be inoculated with smallpox in an effort to protect them against the possibility of a virulent infection due to a then-raging epidemic. Abigail Adams to John Adams, July 13–14, 1776, *Adams Family Papers: An Electronic Archive*, Massachusetts Historical Society, www.masshist.org/digitaladams/aea/cfm/doc.cfm?id=L17760713aa.

4. See the World Health Organization at www.who.int/csr/don/2013_07_15/en/ and www.emro.who.int/polio/polio-news/new-polio-virus-egypt.html. The site www.polioeradication.org describes the latest efforts in the eradication campaign. A map can be seen at www.polioeradication.org/Dataandmonitoring.aspx.

5. M. Feldmann and R. N. Maini, "Anti-TNF Alpha Therapy of Rheumatoid Arthritis: What Have We Learned?" *Annual Review of Immunology* 19 (2001): 163–96.

6. The organism has now been renamed *Pneumocystis jiroveci*.

7. M. Worobey, M. Gemmel, D. E. Teuwen, et al. "Direct Evidence of Extensive Diversity of HIV-1 in Kinshasa by 1960," *Nature* 455 (2008): 661–64.

Chapter 3. The Laws of Immunology

1. I was fortunate to work in Av Mitchison's laboratory years later when he was a leading researcher at the National Institute for Medical Research in London, and I came to know and admire him. Av had a most interesting background. His father was an important Labor politician who became a life peer, and his mother, Naomi Mitchison, was a renowned author. James Watson, the co-discoverer of the structure of DNA, describes visits to the Mitchisons in *The Double Helix* (New York: Atheneum, 1968), which is dedicated to Naomi Mitchison. Av's uncle was the famous British geneticist J. B. S. Haldane, and Av claimed to have an ancestor named Napier who is credited with the invention of logarithms.

2. This is another oversimplification. Recent work has shown that helper T cells have many important functions, which I discuss later. A subpopulation of Th cells, designated T follicular helper cells, or Tfh cells, carry out the process of aiding B cells to develop into antibody-producing cells.

3. To be more precise, the term for a molecule that elicits an immune response is an *immunogen*. The immunogen bears chemical structures for which the response is specific, structures termed *antigenic determinants*. The term *antigen* is a general term that often subsumes both meanings.

Chapter 4. Growing Up and Learning Immunology

1. Of course, it is an oxymoron to speak of truth and experimental science. What we have is a construction that best fits the available facts and that is subject to change or "improvement" as we continue to learn more. This is of course a very unsophisticated version of Popper's principle of falsifiability lying at the heart of useful knowledge in the fields of science.

2. A. S. Cohen and W. E. Paul, "Relationship of Gamma-Globulin to the Fibrils of Secondary Human Amyloid," *Nature* 197 (1963): 193–94; W. E. Paul and A. S. Cohen, "Electron Microscopic Studies of Amyloid Fibrils with Ferritin Conjugated Antibody," *American Journal of Pathology* 43 (1963): 721–38.

3. J. L. Goldstein and M. S. Brown, "History of Science: A Golden Era of Nobel Laureates," *Science* 338 (2012): 1033–34. Michael Brown and Joseph Goldstein themselves shared the 1985 Nobel Prize in Physiology or Medicine "for their discoveries concerning the regulation of cholesterol metabolism."

4. R. S. Yalow and S. A. Berson, "Assay of Plasma Insulin in Human Subjects by Immunological Methods," *Nature* 184 (1959): 1648–49.

5. I first came up to Baruj's laboratory at NYU to be interviewed in 1962, on the Monday of the critical week of the Cuban Missile Crisis, so the visit is deeply ingrained in my memory.

Chapter 5. Vaccines and Serum Therapy

1. The maxim comes from a lecture that Pasteur had given in 1854 at the University of Lille.

2. This organism is actually *Pasteurella multocida* and is not related to *Vibrio cholerae*, the causative agent of human cholera.

3. L. A. Pasteur, "A Summary Account of Experiences at Pouilly-le-Fort, Near Mélun, on Anthrax Vaccination," *Comptes rendus de l'Academie des Science* 92 (1881): 1378–83.

Chapter 6. How Is Specificity Achieved?

1. Ehrlich's remarkable career was chronicled in the 1940 film *Dr. Ehrlich's Magic Bullet*, starring Edward G. Robinson.

Chapter 7. Immunology's "Eureka"

1. N. K. Jerne, "The Natural-Selection Theory of Antibody Formation," *Proceedings of the National Academy of Sciences USA* 41 (1955): 849–57.

2. F. M. Burnet, *The Clonal Selection Theory of Acquired Immunity* (Cambridge: Cambridge University Press, 1959).

3. This, of course, assumes that the likelihood of coproduction of antibodies of any specificity is random.

Chapter 8. How Does Each Lymphocyte Develop a Distinct Receptor?

1. BCRs are a form of antibody specialized to reside in cell membranes and part of a molecular complex capable of transducing biochemical signals in the cell. When I speak of the problem of encoding antibody specificities, it should be understood that I refer as

well to BCRs, but since these are encoded (at least for purposes of specificity) by the same genes, the problem is identical.

2. Of course, I have overdrawn the situation. The structure of antibodies was already known, and they consisted of two chains: heavy (H) chains and light (L) chains. Based on sequence analysis, it was clear that each contributed to the specificity of the antibody they jointly formed. Since there was evidence that H chains and L chains could pair in a quasi-random manner, one could imagine that combinatorial expression of only limited numbers of H chain genes and L chain genes could result in a very large repertoire without necessarily breaking the genome bank.

3. N. Hozumi and S. Tonegawa, "Evidence for Somatic Rearrangement of Immuno-globulin Genes Coding for Variable and Constant Regions," *Proceedings of the National Academy of Sciences of the United States of America* 73 (1976): 3628–32.

4. Actually, some antibodies consist of multiples of this unitary structure.

5. Three-dimensional structures of an antibody molecule bound to antigen have been obtained by X-ray crystallography. These structures show that the $V_H D J_H$ junctional area usually makes direct contact with the antigenic epitope.

6. Indeed, some tumors of lymphocytes (lymphomas and leukemias) display joining of genetic elements derived from immunoglobulins or T-cell receptors with other genetic elements often creating new genes that code for proteins that contribute to the malignancy of the tumor.

Chapter 13. What Is Tolerance?

1. Ray Owen, interviewed by Rachel Preud'homme, October–November 1983, Archives of the California Institute of Technology.

2. R. D. Owen, "Immunogenetic Consequences of Vascular Anastomoses between Bovine Twins," *Science* 102 (1945): 400–401.

3. Mitchison describes in glowing terms his tutorial sessions with Medawar in an oral history interview at www.webofstories.com/play/avrion.mitchison/29.

4. J. W. Uhr, "The 1984 Nobel Prize in Medicine," *Science* 226 (1984): 1025–28.

Chapter 15. Regulatory T Cells and the Prevention of Autoimmunity

1. R. S. Wildin, S. Smyk-Pearson, and A. H. Filipovich, "Clinical and Molecular Features of the Immunodysregulation, Polyendocrinopathy, Enteropathy, X Linked (IPEX) Syndrome," *Journal of Medical Genetics* 39 (2002): 537–45.

Chapter 16. Different Structures, Different Functions

1. Molecular weight is the sum of the atomic weights of all the atoms in a molecule. The weight is expressed as a unit, the *dalton*, named in honor of John Dalton, an English scientist who was a pioneering student of modern atomic theory. The individual components of proteins, the amino acids, vary in their molecular weights from a low of 75 for glycine to a high of 204 for tryptophan. If we assume an average amino acid to weigh about 140 daltons, a molecule of 150,000 daltons would contain about 1,070 amino acids.

2. Papain is an enzyme found in papaya. It catalyzes a chemical reaction that cuts proteins at certain preferred sites.

3. The situation is somewhat more complex, given the two different types of L chains, kappa (κ) and lambda (λ). Both consist of a V_L (actually Vκ or Vλ) and a C_L (Cκ or Cλ) domain. Any individual antibody molecule has only κ or only λ light chains.

Chapter 17. Specific Types of Infections, Specific Types of T-Cell Responses

1. F. P. Heinzel, M. D. Sadick, B. J. Holaday, R. L. Coffman, and R. M. Locksley, "Reciprocal Expression of Interferon Gamma or Interleukin-4 during the Resolution or Progression of Murine Leishmaniasis: Evidence for Expansion of Distinct Helper T Cell Subsets," *Journal of Experimental Medicine* 169 (1989): 59–72.

Chapter 19. CD8 T Cells

1. Charles Armstrong discovered LCMV in 1934. He worked in the Hygienic Laboratory of the US Public Health Service, the immediate progenitor of the National Institutes of Health. Indeed, he initiated a great tradition of virology research at NIH that led to the discovery of many viruses and to the development of antiviral vaccines in NIH laboratories.

Chapter 20. Dendritic Cells

1. Type I interferons (interferons alpha and beta) are structurally related to IFNγ but use a distinct receptor and are not generally produced by T cells. They are important mediators of innate immunity.

Chapter 21. An "Ancient" Immune Response Controls "Modern" Immunity

1. W. E. Paul, "Between Two Centuries: Specificity and Regulation in Immunology," *Journal of Immunology* 139 (1987): 1–6.

2. C. A. Janeway, "Approaching the Asymptote? Evolution and Revolution in Immunology," *Cold Spring Harbor Symposia on Quantitative Biology* 54 part 1 (1989): 1–13.

3. Szent-Györgyi was a Hungarian biochemist who won a Nobel Prize for his highly creative work on the role of vitamin C in cellular respiration.

4. Gram-negative bacteria fail to be stained by gram stain, a popular stain used on tissue and bacterial spreads. The stain detects peptidoglycans, a substance comprised of repeating sugars and amino acids that are present in much greater amounts outside of the cell membrane of "gram-positive" than "gram-negative" bacteria. This difference reflects a central difference in the properties of the two classes of bacteria.

5. Actually more than thirty-six since there is sometimes more than one molecule with the same IL designation. The best example is IL-1, where there are two related molecules, IL-1α and IL-1β.

6. S. Z. Ben-Sasson, J. Hu-Li, J. Quiel, et al., "IL-1 Acts Directly on CD4 T Cells to Enhance Their Antigen-Driven Expansion and Differentiation," *Proceedings of the National Academy of Sciences* 106 (2009): 7119–24.

7. B. Lemaitre, E. Nicolas, L. Michaut, J. M. Reichhart, and J. A. Hoffmann, "The Dorsoventral Regulatory Gene Cassette Spätzle/Toll/Cactus Controls the Potent Antifungal Response in Drosophila Adults," *Cell* 86 (1986): 973.

8. Recall from chapter 1 that antibodies to TNFα are highly effective in the slowing of progression of rheumatoid arthritis and are now the treatment of choice in this disease.

9. Interferons (IFNs) are potent cytokines that have many effects, among them the capacity to induce anti-viral activity in cells. There are two major types of IFNs, type I (mainly IFNα and IFNβ) and type II (IFNγ). Type I IFNs are made by many cell types, including a particular type of DC called a plasmacytoid DC; lymphocytes generally do not make type I IFNs. IFNγ to the contrary is made by lymphocytes, including Th1 CD4 T cells, CD8 T cells and a cell type called natural killer (NK) cells. For more on the latter, see chapter 23.

10. Baruj Benacerraf, with whom I worked at NYU, was of Sephardic descent and suffered from FMF. Sheldon Wolff, a leader in the study of FMF, was the chief of the major clinical research program in the National Institute of Allergy and Infectious Diseases, and was able to successfully treat Baruj with colchicine, at that time the drug of choice for FMF and still the most widely used drug. Baruj and Shelly, as he was known, became fast friends, and when Baruj was awarded the Nobel Prize in 1980, it was Shelly Wolff and his wife, Lila, who accompanied Baruj and Annette Benacerraf to Stockholm.

11. G. Di Prisco, V. Cavaliere, D. Annoscia, et al., "Neonicotinoid Clothianidin Adversely Affects Insect Immunity and Promotes Replication of a Viral Pathogen in Honey Bees," *Proceedings of the National Academy of Sciences* 110 (2013): 18466–71.

12. Alfred Sommer went on to become dean of the Johns Hopkins School of Public Health, succeeding Donald A. Henderson, the man who led the successful effort to eradicate smallpox. Thus, two successive Hopkins deans were responsible for two of the world's greatest public health accomplishments.

Chapter 22. The Microbiome and Innate Immunity

1. Flavell and his colleagues observed that mice that had heightened susceptibility to fatty liver had more intestinal bacteria of the genus *Bacteroides*, which are a type of gram-negative bacteria that grow in the absence of free oxygen (anaerobes).

2. *H. hepaticus* is related to the bacteria *H. pylori*, which is a major cause of stomach ulcers in humans.

Chapter 23. Evolution of the Immune System and Innate Lymphoid Cells

1. K. Kärre, H. G. Ljunggren, G. Piontek, and R. Kiessling, "Selective Rejection of H-2-Deficient Lymphoma Variants Suggests Alternative Immune Defence Strategy," *Nature* 319 (1986): 675–78.

Chapter 24. The HIV Epidemic and the Office of AIDS Research

1. From the OAR website, www.oar.nih.gov/about/history.asp.

2. B. N. Fields, "AIDS: Time to Turn to Basic Science," *Nature* 12 (1994): 95–96.

3. See "Major Report on Aids Research at NIH" (press release, March 14, 1996), http://archive.hhs.gov/news/press/1996pres/960314f.html, and Lawrence K. Altman, "Panel Offers Sharp Criticism of AIDS Research Projects," *New York Times*, March 14, 1996, http://partners.nytimes.com/library/national/science/aids/031496sci-aids.html. Copies of the Levine report can be obtained from the NIH Office of AIDS Research.

4. L. Mofenson, J. Balsley, R. J. Simonds, M. F. Rogers, and R. R. Moseley, "Recommendations of the U.S. Public Health Service Task Force on the Use of Zidovudine to Reduce Perinatal Transmission of Human Immunodeficiency Virus," *Morbidity and Mortality Weekly Report* 43 (1994): 1–15.

Chapter 25. How the Immune System Causes Rheumatoid Arthritis and Lupus

1. HLA refers to the human MHC. The abbreviation means human leukocyte antigen. HLA-A, B, and C encode type I MHC molecules. HLA-DR, DQ, and DP encode type II MHC molecules. There are many alternatives at the loci encoding each type I and type II MHC molecule, which are designated by numbers that follow the gene designation (i.e., HLA-DR4).

2. Citrulline is an amino acid that does not normally appear in proteins. However, there are enzymes that can convert the amino acid arginine into citrulline. Peptides containing this modified amino acid are designated *citrullinated peptides*.

Chapter 28. Can the Immune System Control Cancer?

1. M-H. Chang, C-J. Chen, M-S. Lai, et al., "Universal Hepatitis B Vaccination in Taiwan and the Incidence of Hepatocellular Carcinoma in Children," *New England Journal of Medicine* 336 (1997): 1855–59.

2. R. T. Prehn and J. M. Main, "Immunity to Methylcholanthrene-induced Sarcomas," *Journal of the National Cancer Institute* 18 (1957): 769–78.

Chapter 29. New Parts for Old

1. "An Interview with Dr. Joseph Murray, Organ Transplant Pioneer," *On the Beat* [2004], www.donatelifeny.org/uploaded_files/tinymce/files/interview_joseph_murray.pdf.

2. "60 Lives, 30 Kidneys, All Linked," *New York Times*, February 18, 2012.

3. US Department of Health and Human Services, HRSA, Organ Procurement and Transplantation Network, http://optn.transplant.hrsa.gov/latestData/rptData.asp.

Chapter 30. Julien

1. Information on the award is at http://law2.syr.edu/academics/centers/lch/association_award.html.

Conclusion

1. David Hilbert, "Mathematical Problems," *Bulletin of the American Mathematical Society* 8 (1902): 437–79.

2. Address at the dedication ceremony of the Ryerson Physical Laboratory at the University of Chicago in 1894.

3. Reportedly from an address to the British Association for the Advancement of Science in 1900.

4. J. Ohara and W. E. Paul, "Receptors for B-cell Stimulatory Factor-1 Expressed on Cells of Haematopoietic Lineage," *Nature* 325 (1987): 537–40.

5. S. Wenzel, L. Ford, D. Pearlman, et al., "Dupilumab in Persistent Asthma with Elevated Eosinophil Levels," *New England Journal of Medicine* 368 (2013): 2455–66; "Sanofi and Regeneron Report Positive Proof-of-Concept Data for Dupilumab, an IL-4R alpha Antibody, in Atopic Dermatitis" (March 2, 2013), http://investor.regeneron.com/releasedetail.cfm?releaseid=744703.

6. R. Ravindran, N. Khan, H. I. Nakaya, et al., "Vaccine Activation of the Nutrient Sensor GCN2 in Dendritic Cells Enhances Antigen Presentation," *Science* 343 (2014): 313–17.

Index